E & M Coding
Clear & Simple

Evaluation & Management
Coding Worktext

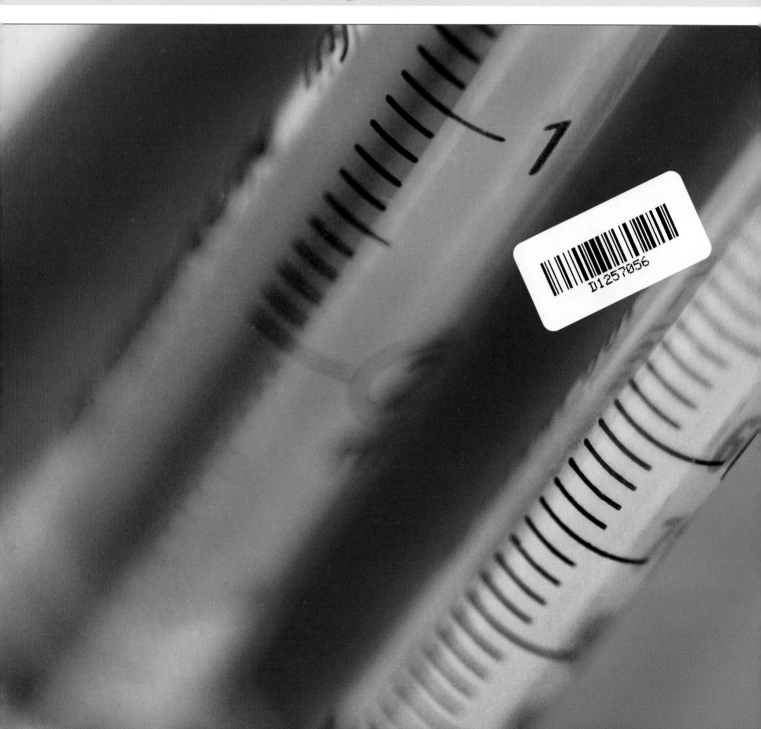

D1257056

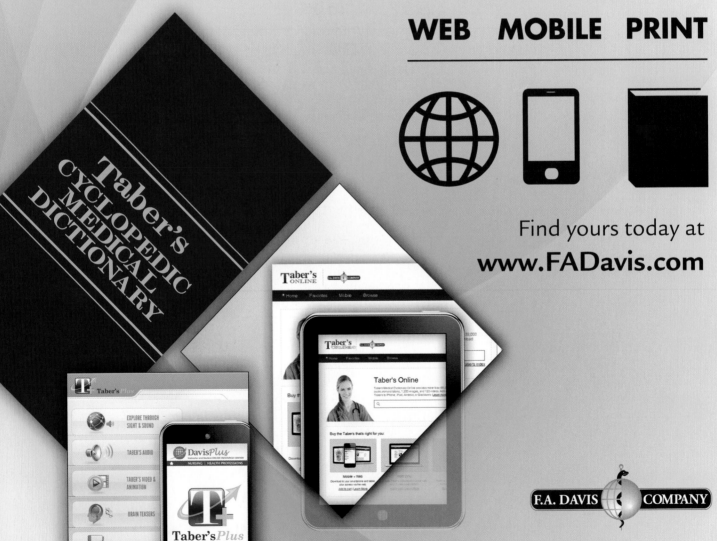

Taber's®
brings meanings to life!

Must-have information... ANYTIME, ANYWHERE.

- FREE, 1-year subscription to Taber's Online
- 33,000 audio pronunciations
- Animations, videos & activities

The choice is yours.

WEB   MOBILE   PRINT

Find yours today at
www.FADavis.com

F.A. DAVIS COMPANY

www.FADavis.com

E & M Coding
Clear & Simple

Evaluation & Management
Coding Worktext

Terri Brame, MBA, CHC, CPC, CGSC, CPC-H, CPC-I

Compliance Education Officer
Institutional Compliance
University of Arkansas for Medical Sciences
Little Rock, Akansas

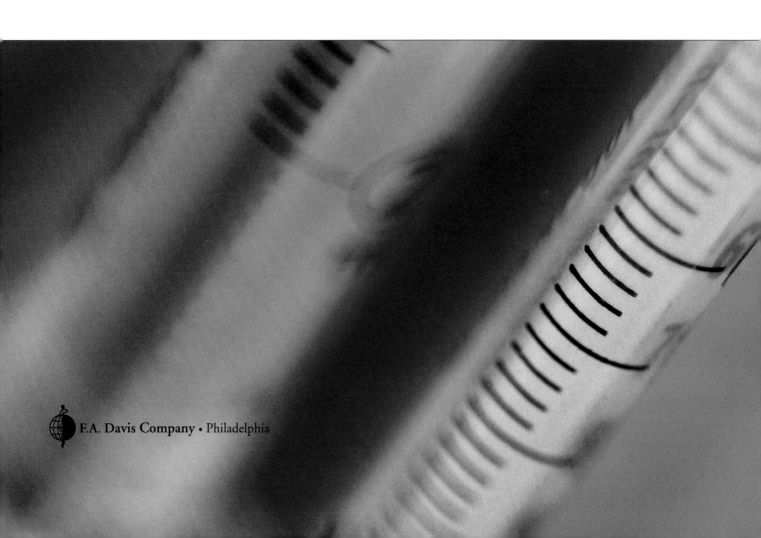

F.A. Davis Company • Philadelphia

F. A. Davis Company
1915 Arch Street
Philadelphia, PA 19103
www.fadavis.com

Copyright © 2014 by F. A. Davis Company

All rights reserved. This product is protected by copyright. No part of it may be reproduced, stored in a retrieval system, or transmitted in any form or by any means, electronic, mechanical, photocopying, recording, or otherwise, without written permission from the publisher.

Printed in the United States of America

Last digit indicates print number: 10 9 8 7 6 5 4 3 2 1

Senior Acquisitions Editor: Andy McPhee
Developmental Editor: Donna Morrissey
Manager of Content Development: George Lang
Art and Design Manager: Carolyn O'Brien

As new scientific information becomes available through basic and clinical research, recommended treatments and drug therapies undergo changes. The author(s) and publisher have done everything possible to make this book accurate, up to date, and in accord with accepted standards at the time of publication. The author(s), editors, and publisher are not responsible for errors or omissions or for consequences from application of the book, and make no warranty, expressed or implied, in regard to the contents of the book. Any practice described in this book should be applied by the reader in accordance with professional standards of care used in regard to the unique circumstances that may apply in each situation. The reader is advised always to check product information (package inserts) for changes and new information regarding dose and contraindications before administering any drug. Caution is especially urged when using new or infrequently ordered drugs.

Authorization to photocopy items for internal or personal use, or the internal or personal use of specific clients, is granted by F. A. Davis Company for users registered with the Copyright Clearance Center (CCC) Transactional Reporting Service, provided that the fee of $.25 per copy is paid directly to CCC, 222 Rosewood Drive, Danvers, MA 01923. For those organizations that have been granted a photocopy license by CCC, a separate system of payment has been arranged. The fee code for users of the Transactional Reporting Service is: 978-0-8036-2559/14 0 + $.25.

To my wonderful husband, Dean,
for supporting this journey.

To my dear friend and mentor, Marcella Bucknam,
for finally wearing me down and convincing me to become a coder.

To my enduring best friend, Leslie Tate,
for always having the coffee on.

Between workshops at a coding conference, I spent time visiting a friend's booth in the exhibition hall. The booth next to hers was occupied by F.A. Davis. As I was perusing their publications, Andy McPhee, who would eventually become my inimitable acquisitions editor, approached me and struck up a conversation. The conversation, which eventually came around to my physician coding and compliance career, also revealed that I loved writing and had once pursued a poetry degree. Andy paused for just a moment, but long enough for me to see the twinkle in his eye. His next question was what textbook did I think was missing from the marketplace, and the idea for this book was born.

E&M Coding Clear & Simple: The Why's

What I thought was missing was a textbook devoted to Evaluation and Management (E&M) coding. E&M codes are the most frequently used physician billing codes, but they are usually allotted just one chapter in a Current Procedure Terminology (CPT) or other coding textbook. An entire text was necessary to adequately explore all aspects of E&M.

As well, I thought we could train coders in E&M coding more effectively by turning that training on its head. E&M learning is usually focused on the details of assigning specific audit points for a specific service level, narrowing the focus to only how the code is assigned. Texts leave little time for explaining *why* that code is selected, thereby leaving the coder unprepared to tackle unfamiliar E&M coding situations. I proposed a book that started with *why* coding is done to provide context for *how* to code, teaching coders not only how to assign E&M codes but how to assign E&M codes using critical thinking.

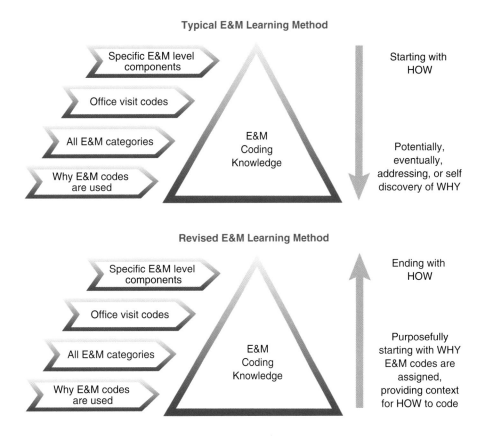

E&M Coding Clear & Simple: The Who's

Instructors with a facility coding background will appreciate the comprehensive nature of this text in addressing a topic that may not be personally familiar. They will also find that the Focus Questions, Critical Thinking questions, and Case Studies are great starting points for class discussion, both in a live setting as well as for online discussion boards. The book is flexible enough to be used as a companion text in a CPT class, as the primary text in an elective course, or as the core text for a program offering a physician coding emphasis.

Students using this text will appreciate the focus on practice and application that will prepare them to code E&M services professionally. I have made an effort to describe each topic thoroughly and methodically so that, as the student progresses into a coding position, the coder will continue to use the textbook as a reference manual for accurate coding. The best way to learn to code E&M services is to practice all elements of coding E&M services, so the student will appreciate the considerable opportunities to apply coding rules to simulated situations.

E&M Coding Clear & Simple: The How's

Throughout the development of this book, I was surprised how much of my process included just sitting and thinking. I thought a lot about why we code E&M services the way we do and how best to share that information.

I also spent considerable time researching source documents for coding rules. I wanted to make sure I identified all source documents accurately. Imagine my surprise when I discovered that all eight elements of the history of present illness (HPI), something used in coding every day, are not included in the CPT manual! As much as possible, this textbook focuses on coding according to CPT guidelines. When the practical method of coding diverges from CPT, such as in using Medicare documentation guidelines, the text also diverges.

In those events where there is really no written rule underscoring a practical coding method or experience, I draw on my personal experience in professional coding and compliance in multiple large academic physician practices and my interactions with government and commercial payers. I have been careful to avoid presenting any information not supported by one of those resources. The Medicare documentation guidelines are included as appendices, and the student should be using the text in conjunction with the CPT manual so that all source documents are readily available for review. Those documents should be read as a student and used throughout the coder's career.

My goals for this book were to teach students both how to code and how to *think* about coding. That approach resulted in the five-part structure, which begins with broad coding concepts and ends with the details of coding a specific visit:

- Introduction to supporting concepts of E&M coding
- CPT manual E&M section that describes all possible E&M codes and service situations
- Levels and components of E&M codes according to CPT
- Medicare documentation rules
- Large coding practice section

FEATURES

The book's features mirror many of the techniques I use to teach E&M coding, especially with the goal of teaching students and coders to think about coding in a critical manner. Instructors will appreciate the Focus Questions, Chapter Summaries, end of chapter Review Questions, and Chapter Case Studies. Those four features will help the student master chapter content.

Students should prepare by reviewing the Focus Questions before reading the chapter. They should read the Chapter Summary to review what they read in the chapter, practice the mechanics of the chapter concept by completing the Review Questions, and apply the chapter concepts to realistic coding scenarios in the Chapter Case Studies. The same clinical scenarios are used throughout the chapter case studies to provide continuity and to review the same situation from different angles.

A coder who understands how to use only Office or Other Outpatient Services E&M codes and how to assign key components for those codes will struggle when the practice adds a hospitalist team, which focuses on inpatient codes. Therefore, most chapters include at least one Critical Thinking question. These questions are open-ended and have no "right" answer. They were designed as classroom or online discussion seeds or even as the basis for short essays. Working on answers to the questions helps the student understand the *why's* of coding.

In actual practice, coders frequently become *de facto* coding instructors for their office. This text supports student coders in developing the ability to teach others about coding—another great way to learn—through Communicating With Medical Providers boxes. Most chapters include a physician-coder communication scenario that most coders end up navigating. The successful coder not only knows how to code but also how to discuss coding with the practice's medical providers. By considering the language being used and the ways in which coding and medical practice may seem, at times, to conflict, coders and providers can avoid common E&M coding issues.

I have written more than 100 case studies and categorized them by beginner, intermediate, and advanced coding levels. I hope that these cases provide the student with an effective way to learn to code E&M services, and the best way to do that is to practice coding. The case studies are based on real coding situations. Medical notes are written in a variety of ways, all of which the student coder will encounter in actual coding positions. The student is provided with a seven-step method for selecting the correct code in any situation.

ANCILLARIES

I include a reproducible audit tool in the textbook and online for use with each Case Study or even in professional practice. The Instructor's Guide includes answers for all seven steps of coding each Case Study, along with rationales for unusual coding situations.

E&M Coding Clear & Simple also includes a comprehensive set of ancillary materials for the instructor and student. The instructor has access to a PowerPoint presentation for every chapter and a comprehensive instructor's guide. Every chapter is accompanied by eight interactive activities on Davis*Plus* (http://davisplus.fadavis.com; keyword: Brame) that may be assigned as homework or used for studying. Activities include key term flash cards, case studies, fill-in-the-blank and multiple-choice exercises, activities to sort terms by category, crossword puzzles, and other items.

FINAL THOUGHT

It has been a long and fascinating journey since that casual booth-to-booth conversation. I hope you will find the outcome as valuable as writing it certainly was to me. *E&M Coding Clear & Simple* is the textbook I wish I had when I was learning to code. And now you can use it to help you enter the remarkable world of E&M coding.

Happy coding!

Terri Ann Brame

ACCREDITING STANDARDS AND COMPETENCIES

Chapters in this book support the following CAAHEP and ABHES standards and competencies. We've listed them here once rather than repeating them in each chapter.

CAAHEP Core Curriculum Standards
VIII. Procedural and Diagnostic Coding

1. Describe how to use the most current procedural coding system

2. Define upcoding and why it should be avoided

VIII. Procedural and Diagnostic Coding

1. Perform procedural coding

VIII. Procedural and Diagnostic Coding

1. Work with physician to achieve the maximum reimbursement

ABHES Competencies

8. Medical Office Business Procedures/Management

t. Coding

u. Insurance claims

y. Effective communication (aa - ll below)

Graduates

 i. Perform billing and collection procedures

 r. Apply third party guidelines

 s. Obtain managed care referrals and pre-certification

 t. Perform diagnostic and procedural coding

 u. Prepare and submit insurance claims

 v. Use physician fee schedule

aa. Are attentive, listen, and learn

cc. Communicate on the recipient's level of comprehension

dd. Serve as liaison between physician and others

gg. Use pertinent medical terminology

hh. Receive, organize, prioritize, and transmit information expediently

 ii. Recognize and respond to verbal and non-verbal communication

kk. Adapt to individualized needs

Reviewers

Ellen Anderson, M.Ad.Ed, RHIA, CCS
  Associate Professor
  Biologic & Health Sciences
  College of Lake County
  Grayslake, Illinois

Marcella Bucknam, CPC, CCS-P, CPC-H, CCS, CPC-P,
COBGYNC, CCC, CPC-I
  Internal Audit Manager
  Chan Healthcare
  Vancouver, Canada

Sheryl S. Chambers
  Certified Billing & Coding Specialist
  Medical Instructor
  Indiana Business College
  Indianapolis, Indiana

Elaine C. Coleman, NCMC, CPC
  MA/General Education Instructor
  Education Department
  ATA Career Education
  Largo, Florida

Deborah Eid, MHA, BA, CBCS
  Instructor/Coordinator
  Portage Lake Career Center
  Adult Education
  Medical Billing and Coding
  Uniontown, Ohio

Eva R. Oltman, MEd, CMA, CPC, EMT
  Professor
  Allied Health/Coding
  Jefferson Community & Technical College
  Louisville, Kentucky

Liza Strickland, BSN, RRT, CPC
  President
  Education Department
  Medical Coding Institute of Texas
  Duncanville, Texas

Jacqueline Thelian, CPC, CPC-I
  Healthcare Consultant
  Medco Consultants, Inc.
  Fresh Meadows, New York

Barbara Tietsort, MEd
  Professor
  Office Information Technology/Medical Assisting
  University of Cincinnati
  Cincinnati, Ohio

Karon G. Walton, AAS
  Program Director
  Medical Assisting & Medical Coding
  Augusta Technical College
  Augusta, Georgia

Acknowledgments

Many thanks to the troop of editors who made this book happen, especially: Andy McPhee, for believing in me; Donna Morrissey, who did more for me in our laughing phone sessions than she knows; Liz Schaefer, who was always ready with an encouraging word; and George Lang, helpful in keeping the technical aspects of the book moving along. Other important people who made this book possible were the reviewers, who took time to critique chapters and offer their insight. Thank you so much for making time in your busy schedules to give me such thoughtful, practical opinions as the book developed. I might have had the idea and created the manuscript, but this book exists due to the efforts of this entire delightful group.

Contents

Introduction to Evaluation and Management Coding

1

History of Evaluation and Management Coding

Chapter Outline

I. E&M Code Origins

II. E&M Defined and Redefined

III. Notes of Interest: What Is and Is Not Covered in This Text

LEARNING OUTCOMES

On completion of this chapter, you will be able to:

1. Understand why Evaluation and Management (E&M) codes are used.
2. Identify the role E&M coding plays in CPT coding.
3. Recognize which aspects of E&M coding are and are not covered in this text.

KEY TERMS

American Medical
  Association (AMA)
Advanced registered
  nurse practitioner
  (ARNP)
Certified nurse-midwife
  (CNM)
Current Procedural
  Terminology (CPT)
Evaluation

Evaluation and
  Management (E&M)
Health Insurance
  Portability and
  Accountability
  Act of 1996 (HIPAA)
Management
Nonphysician practitioner
  (NPP)

Outpatient Prospective
  Payment System
  (OPPS)
Physician assistant (PA)
Procedure
Professional coding
Visit

Evaluation and Management (E&M) coding comprises a small part of the **Current Procedural Terminology (CPT)** but E&M codes are the ones most often used in professional medical coding. E&M coding can be intimidating to a new coder who has heard of the many rules and requirements. This coding is even more difficult for new coders who try to learn it backward by first studying Medicare guideline components and elements, instead of first understanding E&M categories and general rules. This chapter describes the origin of E&M coding, how E&M fits into the CPT scheme, and how this text will cover E&M coding.

⚠ KEY TERMS

CPT (Current Procedural Terminology)—Published annually by the American Medical Association (AMA), including the codes for reporting E&M services.

Focus Questions

Why are E&M codes used to report nonprocedural services?

How does the E&M chapter of CPT differ from other chapters?

How do physicians and facilities use E&M codes differently?

What is compliant coding?

■ E&M CODE ORIGINS

The **American Medical Association (AMA)** published the first edition of CPT in the late 1960s to create a consistent way to describe procedures. It was not until CPT-4 was published in the late 1970s that internal medicine procedures were included, and eventually *visit* (or *levels of service*) codes were introduced. As payers began to use computer systems to process claims, CPT codes became an important part of the medical business; they were a reliable way to report the same service regardless of the provider, region, or payer. Today, CPT is the industry standard for reporting procedures and services and was codified as such as a **HIPAA (Health Insurance Portability and Accountability Act of 1996)** code set.

⚠ KEY TERMS

AMA (American Medical Association)—Publishes the Current Procedural Terminology annually, which includes the codes reported for E&M services.

The original goal of CPT was to codify various procedures and create a consistent way for every physician to report the same procedure. It was much easier to describe procedures, radiological, laboratory, and other testing, because **procedures** were performed in essentially the same way every time and generally described physical actions. Unlike procedures, **visits** have few physical actions and are more concerned with a physician's mental effort. A visit can be completed for many reasons and include several questions and examination elements, depending on the patient's presenting problem and the condition's severity. Visits encompass different work based on the place where the visit occurred. Some visit work is unlike other visit work, such as a visit to obtain preventive medicine versus a visit to have the physician examine a newborn. For many years, CPT did not have a robust method of describing these services, which are unlike services in the other CPT chapters—Anesthesia, Surgery, Radiology, Pathology and Laboratory, and Medicine—but are still so different from one another.

⚠ KEY TERMS

Procedures—Therapeutic or diagnostic actions performed for the patient.
Visit—Involves the physical presence of the patient and the physician's mental effort to evaluate and manage the patient's condition.

In its 1992 annual update of CPT, the AMA scrapped the old way of reporting visits and developed an entirely new chapter of CPT called "Evaluation and Management." CPT 1992 introduced a wider selection of codes to describe services and introduced concepts that are now common concepts such as the seven components, key components, history, examination, and medical decision making. E&M was a new way to describe services that are neither procedures nor tests. **Evaluation** means to determine something systematically. In the medical profession, evaluation usually means to diagnose an illness or injury, including its severity and resolution. **Management** is the treatment of the disease or injury. With regard to a nonprocedural visit, management means to determine the best course of treatment for the patient, order tests, schedule procedures, control drug therapy, and oversee the entire disease process.

KEY TERMS

Evaluation and Management (E&M)—The act of diagnosing and treating an illness or injury, not including performing procedures or tests that can be reported with a CPT code from another chapter.

Evaluation—The physician's effort of forming a systematic opinion about the patient's condition; to determine something systematically.

Management—The physician's effort of determining an appropriate treatment for the patient's condition; the treatment of disease or injury.

E&M DEFINED AND REDEFINED

E&M means diagnosing and treating an illness or injury; the term does not include performing procedures or tests that can be reported with a CPT code from another chapter. Although the work involved in an E&M service can vary widely, it usually falls into similar categories—the seven components of E&M—or is unusual enough to warrant specific codes. These categories can be explained in general terms that can also be more specific in order to describe visits of varying intensity.

Even with the introduction of the E&M chapter and the major overhaul of visit service reporting, E&M coding continues to be a dynamic system. Some codes introduced in 1992 have been deleted, such as Confirmatory Consults and Inpatient Follow-Up Consults. The Critical Care codes receive at least a little revision nearly every year. The goal of CPT and the E&M chapter is to continually refine the description of visit-based services and to represent the current way physicians deliver those services.

Communicating With Medical Providers

Which came first, the code or the service? (Part I)

The AMA created CPT codes to describe services. When those services are E&M visits, coders and physicians sometimes forget that the code describes a service, instead of the service meeting the requirements of a code. Physicians should complete all medically necessary steps of a visit to evaluate and manage a patient's illness or injury. Then the physician should document all of the services performed. Talk with your physician about the difference between medically necessary visit elements and documentation and what must be documented "to get a level." Although it is good to understand what elements are included in an E&M code level, do not let higher codes and potentially higher reimbursement drive up the elements performed in a service or in documentation. Remember that the service came first, not the code.

NOTES OF INTEREST: WHAT IS AND IS NOT COVERED IN THIS TEXT

With the advent of the **Outpatient Prospective Payment System (OPPS)** in the early 2000s, facilities began to use E&M codes to describe the facility portion of outpatient E&M services. Although physicians and facilities use the same code set, the way in which they use the codes and select levels is very different. For that reason, this text focuses on **professional coding**—the coding used for health care professionals rather than for facilities. This is especially important in the later chapters that describe how to select a visit level, because determining the visit level for the work of the health care professional follows a different process than billing for a facility.

❗ KEY TERMS

OPPS (Outpatient Prospective Payment System)—Medicare reimburses hospital facilities for outpatient services based on this system.

Professional coding—The practice of determining the appropriate codes to report services rendered by health care professionals rather than by facilities.

CRITICAL THINKING

> If professionals and facilities use the same code set to describe outpatient E&M services, why would they use them in different ways? What makes professional E&M services and facility E&M services different?

Throughout this book, health care professionals who can bill independently for their services are referred to as *physicians*. However, unless CPT specifically reserves the codes for physician use, *physician* also means any **nonphysician practitioner (NPP)**, such as an **advanced registered nurse practitioner (ARNP)**, a **physician assistant (PA)**, or a **certified nurse-midwife (CNM)**. CPT also refers to these providers as Qualified Health Care Providers (QHPs). As much as possible, CPT attempts to refer to both physicians and QHPs when applicable. Laws vary from state to state on who may bill for services independently, so it is important to understand applicable state law.

Physician is also the preferred term because, although some E&M codes may be reported for all independent practitioners, only physicians may report every E&M code, without regard to specialty. Remember that reporting emergency services is not limited to Emergency Department physicians, nor is reporting newborn critical care limited to neonatologists. As long as the physician is credentialed to perform the service in question, he or she may report the service code.

❗ KEY TERMS

NPP (nonphysician practitioner)—A medical provider who is licensed to bill independently to some extent but is not a physician. Examples are an ARNP, PA, and CNM (synonymous with QHP).

ARNP (advanced registered nurse practitioner)—A registered nurse with advanced training who may see patients independently with a collaborating physician agreement.

PA (physician assistant)—May see patients and bill as part of a physician practice.

CNM (certified nurse midwife)—A nurse with advanced training in midwifery, including prenatal care, delivery, and postnatal care of both mother and baby.

Finally, remember that this text covers E&M coding requirements as defined by CPT. The only reference made to payer-specific coding and billing rules is in the introduction to Medicare Documentation Guidelines in Part 4, because those guidelines are the industry standard. Compliant coding does not mean just following CPT and Medicare rules but also following the rules of every payer. When the written policies of a payer include rules that differ from CPT, they must be followed. Because payer rules can vary so widely, they are not generally addressed in this text.

●●● SUMMARY

- E&M chapter of CPT introduced in 1992.
- Procedure and testing codes describe services consisting mostly of physical actions.
- E&M codes describe services consisting mostly of mental actions.
- Within this text, *physician* means any independent health care professional.
- Facility code level selection is not included in this text.
- Compliant coding requires following the rules of every payer, not just Medicare.

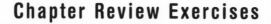

Chapter Review Exercises

1. How many editions of CPT has the AMA published?

2. How often does the AMA update CPT level I codes?

3. What year did the AMA introduce the E&M chapter of CPT?

4. Review CPT procedure code 10060, and list the actions it represents. Determine whether those are physical or mental actions.

5. Review CPT diagnostic testing code 71020, and list the actions it represents. Determine whether those are physical or mental actions.

6. Review CPT E&M code 99221, and list the actions it represents. Determine whether those are physical or mental actions.

7. Compare the three codes you selected in 4, 5, and 6, and describe how they are alike and how they are different.

8. Research whether your state law allows physician assistants to bill independently for services.

9. What is the difference between evaluation and management?

10. What types of physicians may report code 99284?

CASE STUDY

Dawn has started coding in a family practice office where she has been a receptionist for 2 years. She is excited to take on additional responsibilities in the office and wants to understand the coding performed there. In Dawn's situation, answer the following:

1. What chapters of CPT does the office employ?

2. If one of the practice physicians sees a young patient for a school physical, Dawn should select a code from what chapter of CPT?

3. When one of the practice physicians treats a patient with examination and decision making and then excises a mole from the patient's arm, Dawn should select a code from what chapter(s) of CPT?

4. Sometimes, one of the physicians sees a patient at the local Emergency Department. Should Dawn code for the physician's service, the facility service, or both?

5. A hospital coder calls Dawn to see what E&M code(s) she selected in Question 3. Can the hospital coder use the same E&M code for the facility service that Dawn selected for the physician's service?

Evaluation and Management Coding Foundations

Chapter Outline
I. Required Documentation and How to Interpret It
II. E&M Code Frequency

LEARNING OUTCOMES

On completion of this chapter, you will be able to:

1. Describe how documentation is used to develop a corresponding Evaluation and Management (E&M) code.
2. Identify how many E&M codes may be applied on one date of service.
3. Determine when a code should not be reported.
4. Recognize different coding methods.

KEY TERMS

Global surgical package	One Rule	Surgical package
Medicare Physician Fee Schedule Database (MPFSDB)	Presenting problem	

There are a few rules that always apply to Evaluation and Management (E&M) coding. Understanding and applying these rules consistently will help when documentation or correct coding is unclear. These rules consist of the following:

■ What must be documented

■ How often to code

■ When not to code

■ Which coding method to use

Focus Questions

If it was not documented, but *everyone* knows it was done, is it coded?

Can a physician, nurse, or other medical professional who is coding make assumptions about the documentation?

How many E&M codes are assigned when one physician sees a patient twice on the same day?

If a postoperative visit cannot be reported separately from the surgical package, does that mean the service must be provided for free?

■ REQUIRED DOCUMENTATION AND HOW TO INTERPRET IT

The first rule of E&M coding is: *If it was not documented, it was not done.*

All work performed during an E&M service must be documented for patient safety and medical care continuity. Additionally, all portions of a service that a provider wishes to consider when developing an E&M code must be documented. Nothing can be assumed, even if "it is standard practice" or "everyone in my field knows I completed that for this condition" or "I always do that during these visits." Everyone should use written documentation to treat a patient, to bill a service, or to defend a case in court.

 CRITICAL THINKING

What other reasons are there for considering only the written record when coding an E&M service?

✳ Communicating With Medical Providers

Which came first, the code or the service? (Part II)

Along with the suggestions in Chapter 1, another way to discuss correct documentation with a physician is to emphasize using the medical record in patient care. Primarily, multiple providers use a piece of documentation to treat a patient, or a single physician uses the documentation to recall past treatment for a patient. A provider reading complete documentation does not need to guess, assume, or infer to get a good picture of the patient's treatment and condition. However, be clear with the provider that you are not making recommendations on how to document patient care from a medical perspective. Your specialty is coding, and those are the only recommendations you can make. Ideally, your recommendations overlap with good patient care documentation principles. If you are recommending more documentation than the provider says is necessary to treat the patient properly, then the code level you are recommending—or the physician wants to bill—may be higher than is warranted by the medical necessity for the visit. Remember to keep the conversation a dialogue. You and the provider both have valuable input to the discussion. Documentation can also be used for a variety of legal actions. If the documentation accurately represents the care provided and the E&M code reported, it is probably also a good legal document, but that should be left to a legal professional to determine.

In addition to coding only from the written documentation, coders must refrain from inferring any information from the documentation. The most common mistake is assigning a diagnosis code based on a lab value, such as diagnosing renal failure because of increased urea and creatinine levels. If the physician does not provide a diagnosis, the coder cannot assign one. It can be especially difficult for medical professionals to follow this rule when they are coding. For example, physicians coding their own services and nurses who also code are prone to this mistake.

■ Examples of assumed and inferred documentation the provider did not write

- Always giving a point for location in History of Present Illness, assuming the physician always asks the question.
- Inferring that the physician listened to the heart because the physician documented the lungs as clear to auscultation.
- Inferring that the physician ordered certain tests based on the patient's presenting problem.

> ### Examples of assumed and inferred documentation the provider did not write—cont'd
>
> - Inferring a patient has heart failure because the physician notes a low ejection fraction.
> - Assuming that, because the physician marked a certain code on the superbill, the physician spent at least the minimum time necessary to report that code, even though no time was documented in the note.
> - When the physician is seeing a patient in the hospital and has submitted notes for days 1, 2, and 4, assuming a note was written for day 3 and reporting a similar code as those used for the other days.

Coders also stray from the documentation by attempting to decide what work is medically necessary for a patient's **presenting problem**—the reason for the visit—or any resulting diagnosis. For example, if a patient presents with indigestion and as part of the physical exam the physician examines the patient's ears, which does not seem to be related to indigestion, a coder must still consider the ear exam as part of the visit exam. Only physicians may determine what constitutes a medically necessary exam for any presenting problem. If an item is documented, it generally counts toward the code requirements. If the coder has any doubts, the coder should query the physician.

! KEY TERM

Presenting problem—The reason for the visit.

Unless there is physical evidence to the contrary, physician documentation is always assumed to be true and correct. If a physician documents 40 minutes with the patient, the assumption is that the physician spent 40 minutes with the patient. Some coders may want to discount some element of the documentation due to their own disbelief or some assumption regarding the patient's condition. For example, the coder might be surprised that the physician spent 40 minutes discussing a small hand wart that is treated with over-the-counter medication. Unless the coder is also a trained medical professional and is specifically reviewing the note for medical necessity, such as to determine coverage, the coder should not make any coding decisions based on personal opinion regarding whether documentation is accurate. If the coder has a serious concern about accuracy, especially if it affects patient care, then the coder should consult a compliance professional.

■ E&M CODE FREQUENCY

With exceptions (to be described in later chapters), each provider who sees a patient reports only one E&M code for each date of service. This is the **One Rule**—one physician, one code, one day. A physician might see a patient in the hospital on morning rounds and again in the afternoon to check the patient's progress on a new medication. Develop one E&M code for the services provided at both visits on that day. However, the physician might see the patient in multiple places of service on the same day, such as in the office and then later in the hospital. In that case, there are two types of E&M services that the physician has rendered. Later chapters explain how to choose the correct service for the date of service, but only one code is reported for the day.

Sometimes a physician provides an E&M service, but it is not appropriate to report a code. This usually occurs when the E&M service is reported as part of a **surgical package** (also called the **global surgical package).** When surgery or another major procedure is performed, the Current Procedural Terminology (CPT) code reported for the surgery includes the surgery and the package of services covering all relevant elements of the surgery, such as writing orders and immediate postoperative care.

❗ KEY TERMS

One Rule—With some exceptions, each provider who sees a patient reports only one E&M code for each date of service: one physician, one code, one day.

Surgical package/global surgical package—When a surgery or other major procedure is performed, the CPT code reported for the surgery refers to both the surgery and the package of services covering all the relevant elements of the surgery, such as local anesthesia and immediate postoperative care.

Sometimes an E&M service that occurs during the surgical package may be reported separately. Those instances must be reported with a modifier and are discussed in Chapter 3.

 CRITICAL THINKING

Why does it make sense to report a package of services with the surgical CPT code instead of reporting each service on its own?

The surgical package includes a preoperative visit the day of or day before surgery to complete the patient's history and physical. According to CPT, the surgical package also includes all normal postoperative care in the hospital and in the office. As long as the E&M visit is for normal postoperative care, it should not be separately reported from the surgical code. For example, one postoperative visit in the office 10 days after the surgery might be required to follow up on a simple procedure, or monthly visits for a year could be normal for a complex procedure. CPT has considered what is typical *for that procedure* and includes all normal care in building the code. Read the complete surgical package guidelines in the CPT Surgery chapter guidelines.

It is useful here to discuss payer-specific rules. Medicare makes two significant changes to the surgical package. First, it alters the postoperative care contained in the surgical package by also including E&M care provided to treat complications. Medicare also defines the postoperative period by numbers of days—0, 10, or 90, depending on whether the procedure is minor or major. Medicare defines these postoperative periods by CPT code and lists them in the **Medicare Physician Fee Schedule Database (MPFSDB).** It is important to understand which surgical package definition the payer employs before reporting an E&M service.

❗ KEY TERM

Medicare Physician Fee Schedule Database (MPFSDB)—MPFSDB provides the information used by Medicare as a basis to determine payment. The file contains the associated relative value units, a fee schedule status indicator, and modifiers.

Examples of Medicare postoperative periods by CPT code

CPT Code	Description	Postoperative Period Length, in Days
10060	Drainage of skin abscess	10
12032	Intermediate wound repair	10
20600	Small joint injection	0
27130	Total hip arthroplasty	90
31239	Dacryocystorhinostomy, endoscopic	10
32551	Insertion of chest tube	0
49000	Exploratory laparotomy	90
59000	Diagnostic amniocentesis	0
66982	Cataract surgery, complex	90
69210	Remove impacted earwax	0

Find the entire database at www.cms.gov/PFSlookup/

Answer the questions in Figure 2-1 to determine whether an E&M service has already been reported as part of the surgical package.

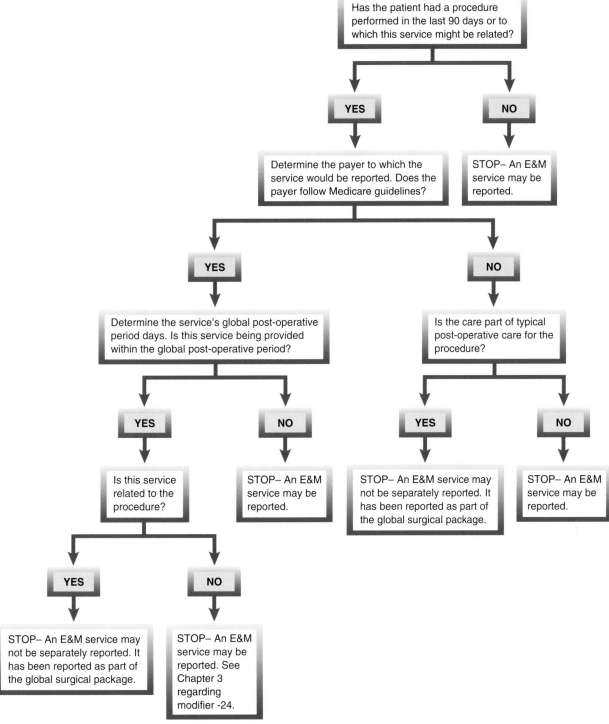

FIGURE 2-1 Algorithm to determine whether an E&M service may be reported.

● ● ● S U M M A R Y

- If it was not documented, it was not done.
- Never assume, interpret, or infer from the documentation.
- One Rule: One physician, one code, one date of service.
- The CPT surgical package includes E&M services for one preoperative visit and typical postoperative care.
- Medicare includes nonoperative complication care in the surgical package and sets the postoperative period at 0, 10, or 90 days.

Chapter Review Exercises

1. If a physician sees a patient in the patient's home and then sees the patient later that evening in the Emergency Department, how many E&M codes should the physician report for that date of service?

2. If a physician sees a patient on hospital rounds in the morning, and the floor nurse calls the physician to see the patient again in the afternoon, how many E&M codes should the physician report for that date of service?

3. When a patient comes into the office for a blood pressure check every day for 5 days, how many E&M codes should the physician report for that week?

4. A patient presents to the office for a scheduled visit for a sore throat, and the physician determines the patient is too ill with chest pains to return home and should be admitted to the hospital. The hospital has a policy that all patients sent for an urgent admission be seen in the Emergency Department, so the physician meets the patient at the Emergency Department to manage the admission. Later that day, the physician stops by the patient's room to check on whether the medication that was ordered was effective. How many E&M codes should the physician report for that date of service?

5. A patient with high anxiety regarding possible illness sets up a series of appointments with multiple physicians on Wednesday. The patient sees an endocrinologist, a neurologist, a urologist, an internist, and a psychiatrist, each for a different presenting problem. How many E&M codes should be reported in total for Wednesday?

For the following questions, determine whether the E&M service can be reported. If you are unable to determine whether a service can be reported, state why.

6. A patient presents with a 4-day history of fever, sore throat, and postnasal drip. The patient has not had any medical care for 1 year.

7. A patient is seen in the office 5 days after having a melanoma removed from her cheek in order to evaluate how the site is healing. The patient is a Medicare beneficiary, and the global period for the surgery is 10 days.

8. A Medicare beneficiary who had total knee replacement surgery sees his surgeon 55 days after discharge. The presenting problem for the current visit is a resolving infection in the knee that has complicated the healing process.

9. A patient who had total knee replacement surgery sees his surgeon 55 days after discharge. The presenting problem for the current visit is a resolving infection in the knee that has complicated the healing process. The patient has commercial insurance that uses the CPT definition of the surgical package.

10. A Medicare patient presents to the office with complaints that her surgical scar is painful and tight. It has been 30 days since the physician performed the procedure.

CASE STUDY

Read this scenario and answer the questions that follow. Explain your answers.

A patient visits a nephrologist regarding recurrent kidney pain. The nephrologist's note reads:

Chris Jones presents with a 2-year history of recurrent kidney pain. The pain has sometimes been diagnosed as kidney stones but with little or no subsequent stone passage. The pain starts gradually and becomes constant, sometimes lasting for 3 or 4 days. It will occasionally radiate into the patient's back and down the thighs. At its worst, the patient rates the pain 8/10 and must take Vicodin to ease the symptoms. Chris has not noticed any problems voiding, and voiding does not increase or decrease the symptoms.

The patient is a plumber and frequently must carry heavy loads and crawl around under houses or in tight spaces. The patient has no family history of kidney cancer, kidney stones, or other urologic conditions.

Vital signs are stable. The patient is resting easily on the exam table. Head & Neck: Normocephalic, PERRLA, EOM, mucous membranes moist and pink. Cardiovascular: RRR, no murmur. Respiratory: Clear. GI: Abdomen soft, no organomegaly, positive bowel sounds. GU: The patient is tender to pressure bilaterally on flanks over kidneys, more on the right than the left. External genitalia normal.

The patient has not had a CT performed for at least a year. Will send for CT and return for follow-up.

1. The physician wants to bill for a consult but did not document the consult requirements. He reasons that because he is a specialist, everyone knows that all of his new patients are consultation visits. Is this a new patient or a consult patient?

2. The physician wants to bill a high-level E&M service that requires a comprehensive physical examination, but he documented only a detailed exam. The physician points out the documentation header "Head and Neck," which means he examined the neck lymph nodes. Because nothing was noted, it can be assumed there was no lymphadenopathy. Documentation of the lymphatic system would qualify the exam as comprehensive. Can the lymphatic system be counted?

3. Can the coder report the diagnosis code for pyelonephritis?

4. The coder is also a nurse and has seen the CT results. She can tell the patient has pyelonephritis. Can she report the diagnosis code for pyelonephritis?

5. In this sort of case, it is standard to schedule lab work. The coder assumes the physician meant to document it and thinks the clinic sent a specimen to the lab. Can the lab work be counted toward the E&M service level?

CASE STUDY—cont'd

6. Consider that the physician's note did include documentation that the patient had no neck lymphadenopathy. The coder does not think the neck lymph nodes pertain to kidney pain and does not think the exam element should be counted toward the E&M service level. This results in a lower-level service being coded. Should the lymphatic system exam be counted?

7. The coder knows that the physician left for the afternoon before the time noted on this patient's chart. The visit note exists, orders were written for the CT, and a follow-up appointment is scheduled, so the patient saw someone in the practice that day. Should the coder report the service?

CPT Modifiers for Evaluation and Management Coding

Chapter Outline

LEARNING OUTCOMES

On completion of this chapter, you will be able to:

1. Identify all CPT modifiers that apply to Evaluation and Management (E&M) coding.
2. Understand the global surgical package and how modifiers split the package.
3. Recognize when it is appropriate to bill separately for E&M services on the same day as a procedure.
4. Distinguish E&M services that are provided for underlying or unrelated services during the global period.
5. Assign the correct modifier to report a mandated service.

KEY TERMS

Global surgical package	Practice group	Underlying condition
Modifiers	Preexisting condition	

Modifiers are an essential part of the information reported for an Evaluation and Management (E&M) service. Modifiers further describe an E&M service that has been altered due to the situation in which the services were provided, but modifiers do not change the definition of the underlying CPT code.

! KEY TERM

Modifiers—Modifiers further describe an E/M service that has been altered due to the situation in which the services were provided, but modifiers do not change the definition of the underlying CPT code.

This chapter describes the CPT modifiers that affect professional E&M services. These modifiers include:

- ■ -24, Unrelated Evaluation and Management Service by the Same Physician During a Post-operative Period
- ■ -25, Significant and Separately Identifiable Evaluation and Management Service by the Same Physician on the Same Day of the Procedure or Other Service
- ■ -57, Decision for Surgery
- ■ -55, Postoperative Management Only
- ■ -56, Preoperative Management Only
- ■ -32, Mandated Services

This chapter also discusses modifier -54 Surgical Care Only, which is a procedural modifier that may be used in conjunction with modifiers -55 and -56.

Focus Questions

When are modifiers appropriate for E&M services?

What are the three major parts of the global surgical package?

Why does an E&M service on the same date of a procedure require a modifier to be reported?

When are E&M services not reported with E&M service CPT codes?

■ MODIFIER CONCEPTS REVIEW

Of the two types of Level I (CPT) modifiers—informational and those that affect payment—all of the E&M service modifiers are the second type; they affect payment. More specifically, they allow full payment of the associated E&M service CPT code, rather than increasing or decreasing the payment amount. Except for -32 Mandated Services, all of the E&M service modifiers allow the reported E&M service to be appropriately reimbursed separately from a global surgical package.

Two coding concepts are important to keep in mind when applying modifiers to E&M services. First, remember that payers consider all providers in the same specialty **practice group** to be the same billing provider when it comes to payment. Therefore, any guidelines referring to a physician also apply to a physician's specialty practice group. This chapter will describe how to use modifiers in the same way—the rules that refer to a physician also apply to the physician's specialty practice group.

Second, while modifiers describe an unusual situation in which the E&M service was provided, the underlying CPT code for the service must still accurately represent the service performed. The modifier does not change the nature of the CPT code.

! KEY TERM

Practice group—Payers consider all providers in the same specialty practice group to be one entity when it comes to payment.

Finally, since many of these modifiers describe work performed in the postoperative period, a brief review of the **global surgical package** is in order. When reporting a surgical CPT code, the code not only describes the operation, but the entire suite of services typically provided for that surgery. This includes a preoperative history and physical (H&P) visit, the operation, and postoperative services directly related to the procedure. Since reimbursement for all of these services is packaged, other services reported during the same period must be described as outside of the package to receive proper payment. The global surgical package is described in the CPT Surgery section guidelines.

! KEY TERM

Global surgical package—When a surgery or other major procedure is performed, the CPT code reported for the surgery
    refers to more than the surgery alone. The surgical CPT code represents an inclusive package of services covering all
    the relevant elements of the surgery, such as local anesthesia and immediate postoperative care.

■ MODIFIER -24, UNRELATED EVALUATION AND MANAGEMENT SERVICE BY THE SAME PHYSICIAN DURING A POSTOPERATIVE PERIOD

As described in its title, modifier -24 is used to report an E&M service that is performed in the postoperative period of a global surgical package where the E&M service is unrelated to the surgery performed. Since it is unrelated, it has not been reimbursed as part of the global surgical package and can be separately reported for payment. There are several circumstances where modifier -24 may be appropriately applied: when treating a **preexisting condition,** when treating an **underlying condition,** and when treating an unrelated condition.

Understanding the global surgical package is vital to properly applying modifier -24, because the package only applies to the surgery—not necessarily to the disease process that necessitated the surgery. Treating preexisting and underlying conditions in the postoperative period are separately reportable from the global surgical package.

! KEY TERMS

Preexisting condition—Condition that was present prior to the current treatment.
Underlying condition—Condition that caused need for the treatment but is not resolved by the treatment.

■ Examples of using Modifier -24

- A patient with occluded heart arteries, which is an underlying condition, may require a coronary artery bypass graft procedure. After the procedure, the patient still has the underlying heart disease, and that will continue to be treated. If the surgeon who performs the procedure also treats the heart disease postoperatively, the services are reported with modifier -24.
- The same patient may also need monitoring for preexisting type II diabetes while the patient is in the hospital, and if the same surgeon provides those services, they are reported with -24.
- Again, the same patient with heart disease is discharged in satisfactory health and returns to see the cardiac surgeon in a week in the office for a follow-up. While there, the patient complains of some itching, redness, and scaling on the arm. The surgeon decides to treat the condition, dry skin, with a prescription steroidal cream rather than send the patient to his primary care physician. Report the service rendered to treat the dry skin, which is unrelated to the surgery, with modifier -24.

Medicare, and many other payers, also specifically identifies two instances of conditions to report with modifier -24. A post–organ transplant patient acquires a new condition—the need for immuno-suppression to prevent rejection of the transplanted organ. This is an unrelated condition from the surgery, and services for immunosuppressive management are reported separately. The second condition is critical care for a severely injured or burned patient. Patients with these injuries often require critical care services for the underlying injury in order to prevent loss of life or to preserve major organ function. Even if the surgery performed is to begin skin grafting for burn patients or to treat a damaged organ for a trauma patient, the associated burn or trauma is considered an underlying condition. These services should also be reported with a burn or trauma diagnosis code.

Remember that this is a modifier used in the postoperative period. If a payer, such as Medicare, uses a specific number of days for the postoperative period, then ensure that the postoperative period is still active before applying modifier -24. If the procedure has zero global days or the time period has elapsed, the modifier should not be applied.

MODIFIER -25, SIGNIFICANT AND SEPARATELY IDENTIFIABLE EVALUATION AND MANAGEMENT SERVICE BY THE SAME PHYSICIAN ON THE SAME DAY OF THE PROCEDURE OR OTHER SERVICE

The title of this modifier says it all! Let's break it down, starting at the end—when the completed E&M service occurs on the same date as a procedure or other service. An E&M service might occur on the same day as a minor procedure or on the same day as certain other E&M services.

Those certain E&M services are preventive medicine services and critical care services, which create exceptions to the One Rule (one physician, one code, one day). If a problem-oriented E&M service is provided on the same day as a preventive visit or critical care services, then consider the preventive visit or critical care services as the primary service, and the problem-oriented visit is reported with modifier -25. Conversely, if a preventive medicine visit or critical care services occur on the same day as a procedure, the procedure is the primary service and the preventive visit or critical care services are reported with modifier -25. Part 2 of this text includes more detailed information to help you determine when using modifier -25 is appropriate.

Significant and Separately Identifiable Evaluation and Management Service—if it is documented, isn't an E&M service always significant and separately identifiable? It is identifiable, but not necessarily significant and separate. If the E&M service is reported with a separate diagnosis than the procedure, then there is sufficient documentation to prove the E&M service was significant and separate. For example, if a patient sees a dermatologist to have a lesion excised and has some facial acne evaluated, the dermatologist reports the procedure and E&M service with separate diagnoses. The difficulty arises when the diagnosis code for the procedure or other service and the E&M service are the same.

If the reported diagnosis for the E&M service and the procedure is the same, documentation becomes very important to show that the E&M service is significant and separate. For example, a vascular surgeon who specializes in wound management might assess a patient's blood sugars and adjust diabetic medication on the same day that a lower leg wound, caused by diabetic complications, is débrided and treated with a vacuum dressing. In this case, the E&M service is reported separately because it was performed to manage an underlying condition. Along the same lines, extensive counseling provided at the time of a procedure may also be separately reported. A breast surgeon who performs a needle biopsy in the minor procedure room and then spends 30 minutes discussing the possible outcomes of the biopsy and potential treatment courses, or discusses with the patient multiple treatment options (wait and see versus excision of a suspicious lesion) prior to performing the procedure, would report that as a separate E&M service.

When these situations do not apply, further examination or assessment of the patient beyond the typical care for the procedure is required for the E&M service to be significant. A minor procedure global surgical package includes assessing the anatomic area of the condition and obtaining informed consent. Because this E&M service does not meet the criteria for being significant or separate, modifier -25 may not be applied.

Examples of when Modifier -25 is and is not appropriate for use when the physician performs a minor procedure

- A patient presents to a primary care physician complaining of a crackling noise and reduced hearing in the right ear. The physician inspects the ear, finds impacted cerumen against the tympanum, and removes the cerumen with a cerumen spoon. Because the physician would always inspect the external ear and ear canal when performing this procedure, reimbursement for that evaluation is included in the procedure code for mechanical removal of impacted cerumen (69210). Thus, an E&M service is not significant and separately reportable, as the work would be reported twice.

- In the same scenario, that patient presents with the same complaint. But this time, the physician takes a pertinent history, which includes noting a current medication that can cause balance problems and dizziness, examines the contralateral ear, and rechecks the patient's blood pressure. The physician rules out other causes of the crackling and hearing reduction and determines the problem is impacted cerumen, which is removed with a cerumen spoon. In this instance, the physician evaluated multiple diagnosis and/or treatment options before determining the removal was the best treatment option, so the E&M service is significant and separately reported.

Properly applying modifier -25 can seem daunting since the requirements are somewhat gray. Remember that modifier -25 has been an Office of the Inspector General (OIG) focus for many years, so it is best practice to ensure good supporting documentation exists when it is applied. Figure 3-1 presents a sound method to use in determining whether or not to use modifier -25.

 CRITICAL THINKING

This topic will be described further in Part 2, but for now, consider that a problem-oriented E&M service and a preventive medicine E&M service are provided by the same physician on the same day. In order to report both services, one must have a modifier -25. It is correct to apply the modifier -25 to the problem-oriented service. Why isn't the modifier -25 applied to the preventive medicine service?

■ MODIFIER -57, DECISION FOR SURGERY

Modifier -57 is another modifier that describes an E&M service that can be reported separately even though it was provided during a global surgical package. The global surgical package includes a preoperative E&M service the day before or same day as a major surgery. This is usually the history and physical update required for hospital admission. For a typical elective surgery, a surgeon sees the patient in the office for a visit at some point prior to the surgery and at that time makes the decision for surgery. The surgery is scheduled for a future date and the patient proceeds with preoperative tests and preparation.

However, if the decision for surgery is made the day before or the day of surgery, such as in a trauma situation, that visit is separately reportable. The physician work required to determine a diagnosis and to consider treatment options is not included in the reimbursement for the global surgical package. The documentation should clearly state that the decision for surgery was made at this visit.

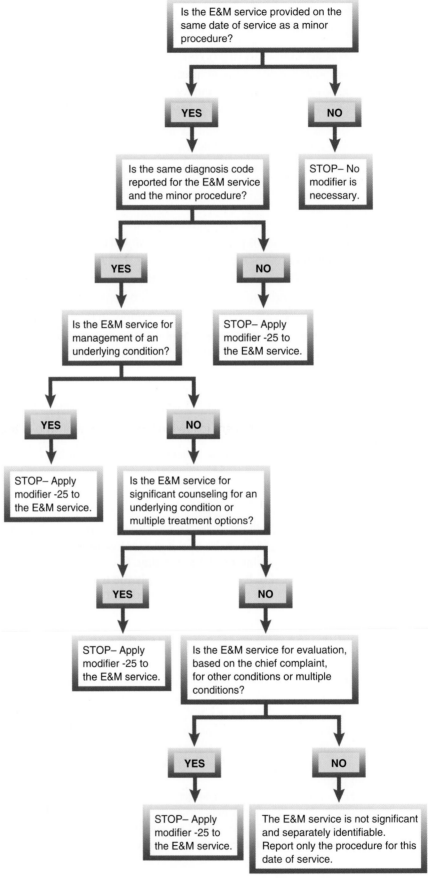

FIGURE 3-1 Modifier -25 decision tree.

■ SPLITTING THE SURGICAL PACKAGE

The global surgical package can be split into three major sections: preoperative, intraoperative, and postoperative care. Usually, the same surgeon (or surgical practice) provides all three sections, and so one surgeon reports the entire package. However, there are occasions when two or more surgeons provide the surgical package. Most commonly, the surgical package is split when a second provider completes the E&M portion of the intraoperative section or all postoperative care.

■ MODIFIER -54, SURGICAL CARE ONLY

Modifier -54 is not an E&M modifier, but it is important to understand how to use it in combination with modifiers -55 and -56 to split the global surgical package. It is also important to understand how to use modifier -54 to report situations where the intraoperative portion is further divided. The surgeon who completes the intraoperative portion of the global surgical package reports modifier -54. The intraoperative portion of the global surgical package includes the operation per se, local anesthetics, writing postoperative orders, and evaluating the patient in the recovery area.

The intraoperative portion of the global surgical package also includes E&M services provided during the remainder of the postoperative hospitalization. If the patient's care is transferred immediately after surgery to another specialty, such as cardiac surgery transferring a patient to cardiology, the physician receiving the patient will report subsequent hospital care codes for the remaining inpatient care.

■ Examples of when to apply Modifier -54

- A postoperative patient following hip replacement who is transferred to a hospitalist service and then to an outside physician for the postoperative period.
- An open-heart surgery patient transferred to a cardiologist staffing the cardiac intensive care unit.
- Patient sent for neurological surgery from the closed trauma ICU is returned to the care of the general surgeon staffing the unit.
- In smaller hospitals, the patient's primary care physician may be responsible for the patient's postoperative care.

■ MODIFIER -55, POSTOPERATIVE MANAGEMENT ONLY

The postoperative portion of the global surgical package starts when the patient is discharged from the hospital. Modifier -55 is reported when care is transferred to a different provider outside of the surgeon's specialty practice group. If multiple providers in the same group provide portions of the global surgical package, the operating surgeon reports the entire package without a modifier.

Modifier -55 is used when a patient travels out of state for a procedure but returns home after surgery. The patient is stabilized immediately postsurgery, and upon discharge is sent home, with a transfer of care to a local surgeon postoperatively. The receiving surgeon *does not* bill E&M codes for the services provided. Instead, the receiving surgeon bills the primary procedure code from the surgery, with modifier -55. The receiving surgeon also uses the surgical date of service.

Example of how to use Modifier -55

A 48-year-old man from northern Louisiana with a 9-month history of abdominal pain travels to Dallas, Texas, for an exploratory laparotomy to determine the source of the pain. The surgery is performed on October 1. The surgical findings are adhesions from an old laparoscopic surgery. The adhesions are lysed. The patient has an uneventful hospital course and is discharged from the hospital postop day 3. Because the patient is far from home and the surgery and diagnosis are uncomplicated, the patient is discharged to the care of the patient's hometown primary care provider (PCP). The PCP sees the patient twice in the postoperative period to monitor wound healing and pain management, without complication. The reported codes for this care are:

Operative surgeon: DOS October 1   CPT 49000-54
PCP: DOS October 1   CPT 49000-55

Although the PCP's services are not performed on October 1, it is appropriate to report the date of service in this manner. Consider if one surgeon performs the entire surgical package—one code is billed on one date, but the services of the three parts of the surgical package are performed on multiple days. By reporting the PCP's services on the date of the surgery rather than the dates the PCP saw the patient, it describes to the payer that the care is related to the surgery.

MODIFIER -56, PREOPERATIVE MANAGEMENT ONLY

Note that the previous example did not include reporting modifier -56. Many carriers, especially Medicare, do not recognize modifier -56, and the modifier is often no longer reported or reimbursed. In practice, first verify with the carrier that it may be reported. Carriers that do not recognize modifier -56 typically consider the preoperative history and physical to be part of the intraoperative care. However, if it is a recognized modifier, the service documentation should clearly show who is providing the care. In rare instances, one physician provides both the preoperative and postoperative care, and the intraoperative care only is provided by a different surgeon. Regardless, services with modifier -56 are reported in the same way—by appending the primary surgical procedure code and using the date of the surgery as the date of service. The following is an example of how to split the surgical package as far as possible for billing purposes.

Example of splitting the surgical package as far as possible for billing purposes

A patient from Stillwater, Oklahoma, travels to Houston, Texas, for an operation. He will arrive the day before surgery and return home as soon as he is discharged.

A general surgeon in Houston, Texas, performs an exploratory laparotomy (49000) on December 1.

The day before, November 30, a physician from the preoperative services department completes the patient's history and physical.

A hospitalist manages the patient's care on December 2, 3, and 4.

The patient is discharged home to Stillwater, Oklahoma, to be followed postoperatively by his family physician.

Example of splitting the surgical package as far as possible for billing purposes—cont'd

Provider	Surgical Package Portion	Actual Date of Service	Reported Date of Service	CPT Code(s)	Modifier
General Surgeon	Intraoperative	12/01	12/01	49000	54
Hospitalist	Intraoperative (inpatient postop care)	12/02–12/04	Actual dates of services	99231–99233	None
Family Physician	Postoperative	12/05–03/02	12/01 (reported once)	49000	55
Preoperative services physician	Preoperative	11/30	12/01	49000	56

CRITICAL THINKING

Why is modifier -56 not recognized? What circumstances might lead Medicare specifically to never allow the preoperative H&P to be reported (think teaching hospitals)?

MODIFIER -32, MANDATED SERVICES

The mandated services modifier -32 may be applied to E&M services as well as procedures. It is assigned when a third party requires the patient to have specific services performed. A Workers Compensation plan might require a second opinion before scheduling surgery. A correctional facility might require a fitness exam. In these instances, there may not be the typical medical necessity for a visit, or it might appear that multiple providers are treating the same condition. Modifier -32 is also used as a signal that someone other than the patient will be responsible for payment. The modifier is not applied when a patient or the patient's family seeks a second opinion, only when a third party initiates care.

CRITICAL THINKING

What are other events that would require -32 to be reported?

E&M modifiers are crucial to proper CPT coding and reporting. They are essential for properly reporting services that are otherwise considered bundled into another reimbursed service or not considered medically necessary. These modifiers affect payment because they allow payment to occur. It is easy to overlook proper reporting and reimbursement for E&M services, especially in a surgical practice that receives the bulk of its revenue from procedures, where most of these modifiers would apply. However, proper E&M service reporting and reimbursement is essential to successful fiscal practice management.

❈ Communicating With Medical Providers

Modifiers often describe exceptional situations when reporting an E&M service outside of the global surgical package. More often, the E&M service in question is not separately reportable. Both physicians and coders fall into the trap of describing that service as "not billable" or saying, "We don't get paid for that." Recall that when a surgical package is developed, it includes the work and reimbursement for many E&M services. Try to change your thinking and the way in which you communicate with physicians, from "not receiving payment for a service" to "not receiving payment *twice*." The service is already reimbursed as part of the surgical package, so it would be inappropriate to report it again. Whether the amount of reimbursement received for the service is adequate is another matter, but encourage your physicians to recognize that the service has been reported and reumbursed.

●●● SUMMARY

- E&M service modifiers affect payment, by allowing payment.
- For reimbursement purposes, all providers in a specialty practice are considered the same billing provider.
- E&M service modifiers describe the situation in which the service is provided but do not alter the underlying CPT code.
- Many E&M service modifiers describe a service that is reportable even though it was performed during a global surgical package period.
- Modifier -24 describes E&M services performed during the global period for underlying or unrelated conditions.
- Modifier -25 describes E&M services performed on the same date as a minor procedure. Refer to the decision tree to determine how to report this service.
- Modifier -57 describes an E&M service on the day of or day before a major surgery that is not the bundled history and physical update but a separate service to consider the patient's diagnosis and treatment options.
- Modifiers -54, -55, and -56 split the global surgical package into intraoperative, postoperative, and preoperative sections.
- The surgical package modifiers always append the primary surgical procedure code, not E&M service codes.
- Always report the surgical package modifiers using the date of surgery, regardless of the date that services are delivered.
- Modifier -56 is often not recognized by payers and the preoperative care is considered part of the reimbursement to the operative surgeon.
- Mandated services, reported with modifier -32, are required by a third party (not the patient, family, or physician) to be performed.

Chapter Review Exercises

Determine the appropriate modifier to apply to each of the following situations:

1. A surgeon who has performed a cholecystectomy for a patient is managing that patient's diabetes while the patient is recovering in the hospital.

2. A surgeon in Billings, Montana, follows a patient's recovery after the patient returns from thyroid surgery in Seattle, Washington.

3. An insurance company requires a patient to receive a second opinion regarding cancer treatment.

4. Before suturing a scalp laceration in the emergency department, the physician examines the patient's psychological and neurological status to determine whether the patient also received a concussion.

5. A gynecological surgeon provides preoperative and intraoperative care for a Medicare patient with ovarian cancer before transferring the patient to a gynecological oncologist. (Determine the modifier for surgeon's services.)

6. A head and neck surgeon performs a tonsillectomy on a 9-year-old girl, and the patient's primary care physician monitors her postoperative healing. (Determine the modifier for surgeon's services.)

7. A hospitalist completes the preoperative history and physical for a patient prior to a scheduled complete knee arthroscopy.

8. While stabilizing a patient in the emergency room following a vehicle collision, the trauma surgeon determines the patient needs emergency exploratory surgery and takes her to the operating room immediately.

9. A surgeon must continue to manage a patient's Crohn's disease in the postoperative period of a partial colectomy.

10. Before offering a customer a product, a life insurance company requires the customer to have a complete physical completed.

CASE STUDY

Assign the correct modifier for each visit.

Henry Kim is a 35-year-old welder in Grand Island, Nebraska. While at work welding, a metal splinter became lodged in Henry's eye. Henry went to the emergency room. Henry complained of pain from the splinter as well as a feeling of light-headedness and shortness of breath. The physician on duty completed a full examination of Henry and determined that his non-pain symptoms were due to hyperventilation secondary to the accident at work. The physician then examined the Henry's eye with a slit lamp and saw the splinter lodged in his cornea. The physician carefully removed the splinter from Henry's eye, bandaged it, and sent him home with aftercare instructions.

1. Select a modifier that applies to this situation for the emergency physician's E&M service.
   As the next few weeks went by, Henry's vision became increasingly blurry, his eye watered continuously, and he continued to experience pain. Henry went to a local ophthalmologist for further treatment. The ophthalmologist determined that the emergency physician did not remove the entire metal splinter from Henry's cornea, likely due to the very small size of the splinter. It was the ophthalmologist's opinion that the cornea had been permanently scarred, and the only treatment that would restore Henry's vision would be a corneal transplant. Because corneal transplants are an expensive treatment, Henry's employer's Workers Compensation insurance carrier wanted him to have a second opinion from an ophthalmologist, who also happened to perform corneal transplants, at the academic medical center in Omaha, Nebraska. Henry traveled to Omaha, about 3 hours away, to see the second ophthalmologist, who agreed that a transplant was necessary.

2. Select a modifier that applies to the Omaha ophthalmologist visit.
   Surprisingly, a cornea donation was available that was a match for Henry, and surgery was scheduled for early the next morning.

3. Select another modifier that should be applied to the Omaha ophthalmologist visit.
   Henry had surgery the next day, and the transplant was a success. Since he was otherwise healthy, the surgeon thought he could recover at home and be followed by the ophthalmologist in Grand Island. To be sure everything was going well, Henry stayed in the hospital overnight and went home the next day.

4. Select a modifier that applies to the surgery.
   Henry saw his ophthalmologist in Grand Island at regular intervals to see how well the graft was healing. Everything looked fine, although the typical postoperative care for a corneal transplant lasts at least a year. During the postoperative period, Henry saw the ophthalmologist for an annual eye health check-up, which was fine.

5. Select a modifier for the postoperative care provided in Grand Island.

6. Select a modifier for the general eye examination.
   Henry's eye eventually healed, and since his eyes were otherwise healthy, his vision returned to normal.

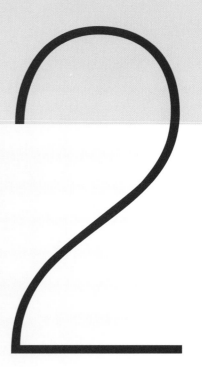

Structure of the Evaluation and Management Section of CPT

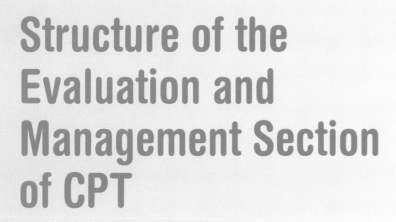

4

Introduction to Evaluation and Management Subsections (Categories)

Chapter Outline

I. E&M Service Guidelines
   A. Classification of E&M Services
   B. Definition of Terms Unique to E&M
   C. Other Guidelines
   D. Instructions for Selecting an E&M Service Level

II. E&M Category Traits
   A. Place of Service
   B. Patient Status
   C. Type of Service
   D. E&M Category Traits Review

LEARNING OUTCOMES

On completion of this chapter, you will be able to:

1. Use the Evaluation and Management section guidelines to support correct code selection.
2. Select correct Evaluation and Management (E&M) categories based on knowledge of the three defining traits.
3. Differentiate between outpatient and inpatient E&M categories.
4. Correctly classify new and established patients.

KEY TERMS

Ambulatory care	Inpatient	Patient status
Consultation	New patient	Place of service
Established patient	Nursing facility	Subcategories
Freestanding	Outpatient	Type of service
Hospital inpatient facility	Oversight services	

The six sections of CPT are large and can vary widely in the types of codes presented. To organize these large sections, CPT further divides them into subsections of varying degree, each with similar structure. This chapter explains the framework of the Evaluation and Management section of CPT and explores how to use the structure of the section to select appropriate codes. The E&M subsections emphasize services provided based on the *place of service,* the *patient's status,* and the *type of service* unique in CPT. Understanding from which E&M subsection, or category, to select a code is the first step to selecting the correct E&M code.

Focus Questions

Is there a difference between an E&M subsection and an E&M category?

How is an E&M category correctly selected?

What are the options for E&M category selection?

In what places do E&M services take place?

What are the two types of patient status?

■ E&M SERVICE GUIDELINES

It may seem remarkable, but the CPT Evaluation and Management section and category guidelines do include all of the information needed to properly select E&M service codes, according to CPT conventions. What is confusing is that the instructions for selecting a level of service are subjective and difficult to apply consistently even with the help of the clinical examples. Because of this, third party payers usually provide additional instructions on how to select a level of service. Fortunately, selecting the correct category and subcategory of E&M service is more straightforward and employs a discrete set of guidelines, which are described in the CPT Evaluation and Management section guidelines.

The CPT Evaluation and Management section guidelines are the largest set of guidelines in CPT. While they include similar topics to the other section guidelines, the CPT Evaluation and Management guidelines include information on the classification of E&M services, instructions for selecting service levels, and the most extensive definitions list of any CPT section. These guidelines are vital to correct coding and apply to all codes in the CPT Evaluation and Management section. Read the entire CPT Evaluation and Management section guidelines together with this chapter.

Classification of E&M Services

E&M categories comprise more exceptions than rules when it comes to structure. It is important to understand how a category *might* be organized to best understand how it *is* organized. For that reason, it is important to be familiar with each category of E&M on its own merit, rather than attempting to apply broad rules to all categories.

CPT divides E&M into over 20 categories, from the sizable Office or Other Outpatient Services to the single code Other Evaluation and Management Services. E&M categories are described in one of three ways: by *place of service, patient status,* or *type of service.* **Place of service** describes the physical location requirement for the services rendered, such as Hospital Inpatient Services. **Patient status** is the patient's physical condition and is the defining aspect of Critical Care Services; or it can be the patient's relationship to the provider, such as whether the patient is a new or an established patient. **Type of service** describes a particular service being provided, such as Consultations.

! KEY TERMS

Place of service—Physical location requirement for the services rendered.
Patient status—The patient's physical condition or the patient's relationship to the provider.
Type of service—A particular service being provided, such as Consultations.

Each of the categories is then arranged in a similar manner. First, categorical guidelines describe when, how, and where the category codes may be used. Similar to section guidelines, category guidelines provide information unique to that category, including what is required to use the category. For example, the guidelines for Office or Other Outpatient Services are rather brief, including information on place of service requirements and direction on how to differentiate outpatient from inpatient status. Guidelines for Critical Care Services are extensive, including unique definitions and bundled services. The guidelines might also provide direction to other categories and reference to the section guidelines.

CPT again uses the terms *subsection* and *category* interchangeably by also describing further divisions of the E&M section as **subcategories.** To avoid confusion, in this textbook we will use the terms *categories* and *subcategories,* except where subsection is the more appropriate term. Many categories are divided into at least two subcategories, which are then divided once more. For example, one common subcategory defines whether a series of codes applies to the patient status: new patient versus established patient. Another common subcategory defines the type of service being provided—initial or subsequent, admission or discharge. Categories might include either one or both of these subcategories.

> **⚠ KEY TERM**
>
> Subcategories—Divisions of an E&M section.

Once the codes are divided into the appropriate categories, the codes themselves are each presented in a similar format, as shown in Figure 4-1. Every code consists of a 5-digit number, beginning with 99, and a description of the service. Next, the *minimum* key components of the service are listed, including history, exam, and medical decision-making. Finally, additional information that applies to the service is listed, such as the general nature of the presenting problem and the typical time spent performing the service.

Many of the categories include related levels of service, which increase in intensity, as with the Subsequent Nursing Facility Care codes (99307–99310). (Review these codes in the CPT manual.) This is a series of four codes, which represent the same type of service, in the same place of service, but increase in intensity based on the severity of the patient's condition and the amount of work

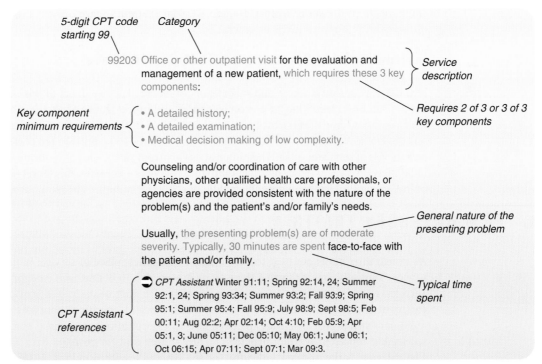

FIGURE 4-1 Copy of code as it appears in CPT.

performed to evaluate or manage that condition. A complete list of E&M categories and subcategories is included at the beginning of the CPT E&M section guidelines.

Definition of Terms Unique to E&M

The Definitions of Commonly Used Terms portion of the E&M section guidelines is the most extensive list of terms in CPT. This glossary is necessary due to the subjective and widely varying nature of E&M. For example, a level three new patient office visit (99203) might be assigned for evaluating dyspepsia and also for managing recurrent low back pain. Evaluating these two problems includes asking a number of different questions, performing significantly different physical exams, and ordering various diagnostic tests. To articulate how both of these visits are assigned to the same code, terminology was developed to describe the basic elements that the visits have in common. These elements and related concepts are defined within the guidelines and constitute many chapters of this text but should be read in their entirety in the E&M section guidelines as well.

Other Guidelines

Unlisted Service is the next topic in the E&M section guidelines and reiterates the CPT guideline on proper use of the E&M unlisted codes. There are two unlisted codes in the E&M section: 99429 Unlisted Preventative Medicine Service, and 99499 Unlisted Evaluation and Management Service. These codes are used when no other E&M service code correctly describes the service provided. This typically applies to emerging services that have not been assigned a category III code or to very unusual services, such as a service provided in an unusual place of service not otherwise listed, perhaps in a place of business.

Unlisted services are supported by documentation in a special report as outlined in the section guidelines. Not only should the special report include an explanation of why the service is being reported with an unlisted code but also should include any other details that describe the service. This might include the length of time spent with the patient, additional tests or services reviewed, special equipment used to provide the service, as well as the typical documentation for any E&M service.

The Clinical Examples Appendix of CPT, Appendix C, is also addressed in the section guidelines. These examples were developed by physicians in various specialties and approved by the CPT Editorial Panel. The examples assist in understanding what effort is required to meet the service levels in different medical and surgical specialties. Each example includes the problem addressed during the service and the specialty that developed the example. The examples are not a definitive source for selecting service levels. Level selection should always be completed based on the components of the specific service rendered. The examples serve only as a guideline and assist in differentiating between levels of service.

Instructions for Selecting an E&M Service Level

The final topic in the E&M section guidelines is selecting the proper level of E&M service. The first step is to select the correct category and subcategory of service. The remainder of this chapter and the balance of Part 2 address identifying the correct categories and subcategories. Once the subcategory is identified, the appropriate level of service must be assigned. Part 3 of this textbook addresses choosing the level of service. Do not attempt to assign the level of service prior to identifying the correct subcategory. How many levels of service exist and their intensities vary from subcategory to subcategory. For example, the middle level, 99203, of Office or Other Outpatient Services describes a shorter service for a milder Nature of Presenting Problem than does the middle level, 99222, of Initial Hospital Care.

■ E&M CATEGORY TRAITS

As noted, three traits are used to define E&M categories: place of service, patient status, or type of service. Typically, one or two of these traits are enough to define each category. Hospital Inpatient Services, which are limited to a specific place of service, represent services provided to patients with a variety of problems. Critical Care Services, which require a specific patient status and type of service, represent services provided in any place of service. Consultations are defined as a specific type of E&M service but represent services provided in any setting and for patients with a variety of problems. The category is the primary indicator for the type of service provided. If the requirements for the category are not met, that category may not be selected.

Place of Service

One of the most important concepts to understand regarding selecting the correct E&M service category is place of service. Many categories and subcategories are defined by the place of service. There are two major types of place of service: outpatient and inpatient. Services provided in transport do not have a defined place of service (Fig. 4-2).

Outpatient

The simplest definition of an **outpatient** is a patient who is specifically not an inpatient in a hospital or nursing facility. The most typical outpatient services, and those most closely associated with the term outpatient, are those performed in physician offices, otherwise known as clinics. Physician offices include primary care clinics, multi-specialty clinics, non-physician provider clinics, community health clinics, and other **freestanding** offices that are not attached to a hospital facility. The services provided in these areas include evaluation and management of illness and injury, preventive medicine services, and special E&M services.

⚠ KEY TERMS
_____

Outpatient—A patient who is specifically not an inpatient in a hospital or nursing facility.
Freestanding—Not attached to a hospital facility.

▮ Examples of outpatient E&M services

- A family medicine physician sees a 42-year-old woman for the first time to discuss headaches that cause nausea.
- Well-child check in an ARNP clinic.
- A baseball player is examined in the emergency department after colliding with another player and briefly losing consciousness.
- A physician sees a patient with terminal lung cancer in her home for pain management.
- A 24-year-old woman is seen in consultation by a surgeon for right upper quadrant pain.

Other outpatient places of service include urgent care clinics that may be free-standing, connected with a physicians' clinic, or attached to an emergency department or other area of a hospital. A patient's dwelling is also an outpatient place of service. There are E&M categories for both the patient's own home and for rest homes, more typically known today as assisted living facilities, which do not provide medical services.

When outpatient care is provided in the hospital setting, it is sometimes called **ambulatory care,** meaning the patient is not confined to the hospital but is able to move about. Outpatient E&M services

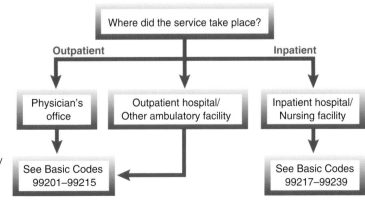

FIGURE 4-2 Identifying category/ subcategory defining traits— place of service.

provided within the hospital include observation status, consultations, emergency department services, short-term care management, E&M provided in ambulatory surgical centers, E&M services provided in hospital based clinics, and other E&M services possibly performed in ancillary service areas of the hospital. In essence, unless the place of service is specifically described as inpatient, it is an outpatient place of service.

❗ KEY TERM

Ambulatory care—Patient receiving services but not confined to the hospital.

Inpatient

In contrast to the wide variety of outpatient places of service, the **inpatient** place of service is very limited and specifically described. Just two places are considered inpatient facilities: hospital inpatient facilities and nursing facilities. These places of service share the qualities of providing room and board to patients while they receive care. While they have separate E&M categories, these places of service share consultation codes.

❗ KEY TERM

Inpatient—Specific admit status to a hospital or nursing facility.

Examples of inpatient E&M services

- A 67-year-old male has an initial assessment performed on inpatient admission for acute kidney failure.
- The pulmonologist caring for a patient's right lobe pneumonia sees her on rounds on the fifth day of an inpatient stay.
- An infectious disease specialist is asked to see a patient with suspicious gangrene of the right foot to determine etiology.
- A nursing home resident with dementia has started falling out of bed at night and is assessed for further mental deterioration.

The difference between hospital inpatient and nursing facilities is whether they provide acute or long-term nursing care. **Hospital inpatient facilities** provide nursing care for patients with acute illness or injury. Hospital inpatient facilities include partial hospital settings for the purpose of E&M category selection. **Nursing facilities** provide care for patients still in need of monitored nursing care but who no longer require care for acute illness or injury. These facilities provide long-term skilled nursing care and rehabilitative services. Nursing facilities include facilities known as skilled nursing facilities (SNFs), intermediate care facilities (ICFs), long-term care facilities (LTCFs), and psychiatric residential treatment centers.

❗ KEY TERMS

Hospital inpatient facilities—Facilities that provide nursing care for patients with acute illness or injury.
Nursing facilities—Facilities that provide care for patients still in need of monitored nursing care but who no longer require care for acute illness or injury.

Transport

Services provided in transport between two places of service are separately identified as neither inpatient nor outpatient. Likewise, they cannot be identified by the places of service between which the transport occurs. Due to the limited nature of professional services provided during transport that are not provided by emergency medical services (EMS) personnel, just three E&M codes address these services:

■ 99288 Physician direction of EMS medical care, advanced life support

■ 99466–99467 Critical care services delivered by a physician, face-to-face, during an interfacility transport of critically ill or critically injured pediatric patient, 24 months of age or younger)

CPT does not include EMS services, which are coded from HCPCS Ambulance Services.

Patient Status

Another way E&M categories are defined is by the patient's status. Patient status includes the status of the relationship the patient has with the service provider or the patient's medical status. Even when not the defining trait for a category, patient status will often define a subcategory and/or affect the level of service selected (Fig. 4-3).

New Versus Established

New patient versus established patient status is one of the primary subcategory definitions. A **new patient** is one who has not received face-to-face services from the provider of the current service within the last 3 years. In contrast, an **established patient** has received services from the physician within the past 3 years. When considering which services have been rendered, any services rendered by the physician, and any other physician in the practice group, are considered. If a physician is covering for another physician, the patient's relationship to the physician who is not available is the one that is considered. For example, Dr. Alexi sees a patient who sees Dr. Makesh every 3 months for a med check because Dr. Makesh is on vacation. A patient who has not been seen in 3 years or more is considered equivalent to a patient who has never been seen because the physician will need to collect the same amount of information in both instances to appropriately evaluate the patient.

❗ KEY TERMS

New patient—A patient who has not received services from the provider of the current service within the last 3 years.
Established patient—A patient who has received services from the physician within the past 3 years.

■ Examples of new versus established patient status

A physician saw all of these patients in a clinic:
- New—A patient last seen 3 years and 2 months ago by the same physician.
- New—A patient last seen 3 years and 2 months ago by another physician in the same practice group.
- Established—A patient seen last year about the same time for a preventive care visit by the same physician.
- Established—A patient seen last year about the same time for a preventive care visit by another physician in the same practice group.
- Established—A patient seen 2 years ago by the same physician but for a different problem than today.
- Established—A patient seen 2 years ago in consultation now presents on his own for evaluation.

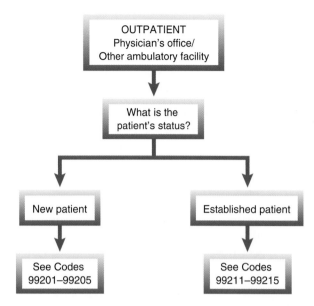

FIGURE 4-3 Identifying category/ subcategory defining traits—place of service/patient status.

Medically Necessary Levels of Care

The patient's condition may also be the defining trait for an E&M category. Sometimes the patient's condition defines what type of care will be provided, making the service medically necessary. The first type of code usually associated with this requirement is Critical Care Services (99291–99296). Critical Care Services code guidelines include a specific definition that must be met in order to use the codes. The key portion of that definition applies to the patient's condition. Continuing Intensive Care Services (99298–99300) require that the patient's condition necessitate a certain level of monitoring.

Another way in which patient condition defines categories is in selecting the correct level of care. If codes are presented in a series, the nature of presenting problem should be met as a minimum to select the correct code. An Office or Other Outpatient Services New Patient visit level 3, 99203, suggests that the patient's presenting problem should be of at least moderate severity to report the code. While the nature of presenting problem is never a required component of an E&M service, it has great influence on code selection and should not be ignored. Comparing a service with the Clinical Examples in CPT Appendix C is helpful in determining the nature of presenting problem.

Examples of medically necessary levels of care

99291—A patient in septic shock must be constantly attended by a physician in order to prevent further deterioration.

99431—A physician physically examines a normal newborn infant after a birthing room delivery.

99479—A low-birth-weight infant requires daily intensive monitoring of his physical status.

99220—Observation status patient who was converted from atrial fibrillation in the emergency department.

Type of Service

Of the three E&M category traits, type of service is the least noticed, but is just as critical when used as the defining trait (Fig. 4-4). As a category-defining trait, Consultations are the most frequently used type of service codes. **Consultation** codes describe the service rendered when a medical professional is asked for an opinion regarding a patient's diagnosis or how best to treat a patient's condition. If a

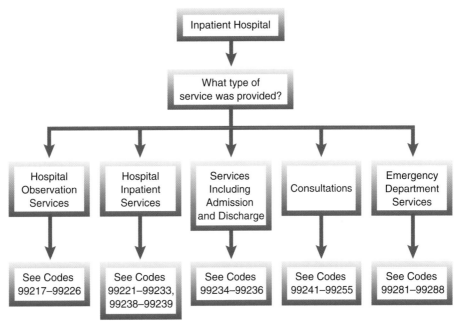

FIGURE 4-4 Identifying category/subcategory defining traits—place of service/type of service.

request for opinion is not made, the service does not apply, making the type of service the defining trait of consultations.

Other types of service codes include various oversight services. **Oversight services** usually take place when the patient is not present. They involve one or more providers involved in the patient's care reviewing data, communicating regarding the patient's condition or care, and making further care decisions. Prolonged services are another type of service codes that have the unique designation of being add-on codes—codes only used along with other codes to describe services that have been provided for a longer than usual amount of time.

! KEY TERMS

Consultation—A medical professional is asked for an opinion regarding a patient's diagnosis or how best to treat a patient's condition.

Oversight services—One or more providers involved in the patient's care reviewing data, communicating regarding the patient's condition or care, and making further care decisions.

E&M Category Traits Review

Whether the category's defining trait is place of service, patient status, or type of service, understanding those traits and how they affect code selection cannot be overemphasized. E&M category traits allow for quick elimination of categories that clearly do not apply to the service in question. A comprehensive understanding of E&M category traits supports appropriate code selection.

❊ Communicating With Medical Providers

Assist your physicians in understanding that the type of provider or specialty where the physician practices does affect the E&M code selected. Rather, it is the quality of the provide service that affects category selection. A psychologist that sees a patient in the emergency department (ED) and is the primary physician for the service may report an ED Services code. Any physician that provides critical care services may report a Critical Care Services code, not just physicians staffing the ICU.

Applying the codes in the E&M section of CPT requires a basic understanding of how to select codes and consideration of what additional information beyond the codes themselves is necessary for proper usage of the section. While good E&M code level selection is the ultimate E&M coding skill, E&M category identification is the true foundation of correct code selection and usage. E&M categories also are the most objective part of choosing the correct code for a service. By embracing these clear divisions within the E&M codes, choosing the E&M category becomes second nature. Building on an understanding of how E&M categories might be structured and comprehending what each E&M category actually represents as well as its particular requirements is the next step in proper E&M code selection.

●●● SUMMARY

- An E&M subsection and an E&M category are the same. The two terms are used interchangeably. Further subheadings under subsections are called subcategories.
- An E&M category is correctly selected by first identifying its defining trait. If the category defining trait does not apply to the service in question, the category is not correct.
- There are three options for determining an E&M category defining trait: place of service, patient status, and type of service.
- Places of service include outpatient, inpatient, and in transport.
- Outpatient is anywhere not specifically noted to be inpatient.
- Inpatient includes hospital inpatient and nursing facilities.
- Transport is neither outpatient nor inpatient.
- The two types of patient status include the patient's relationship to the provider (whether new or established) and the patient's condition and presenting problem severity.

Chapter Review Exercises

1. Name the four primary sections of the Evaluation and Management section guidelines.

2. Inpatient or outpatient place of service—assisted living apartment complex

3. Inpatient or outpatient place of service—hospital cardiac intensive care unit

4. List the two types of patient status.

5. Newborn care services are defined by what trait—place of service or type of service?

6. Identify the correct category for a patient seen in an urgent care center in a shopping center.

7. Identify the correct category for a patient seen in the emergency room. The patient has never been seen at this emergency room before.

8. Identify the correct category for a patient seen by her internist in her home.

9. How many years must pass between visits for a patient to be considered new?

10. If a provider is new to a practice and sees a patient that is established to the practice, for this visit is the patient's status new or established?

CASE STUDY

Identify the defining trait used to select the correct category and subcategory:

John is a 56-year-old long-time patient of Dr. Thompson, an internal medicine specialist. John has a family history of heart disease. Over the past couple of months, John has been experiencing what he thinks is severe heartburn, although his wife has noticed that the heartburn doesn't necessarily coincide with meals. She finally convinces him to go and see Dr. Thompson, if for no other reason than to allay her worries. John sees Dr. Thompson at his clinic, where he practices with seven other physicians. This is John's first visit to see Dr. Thompson in years. He can't remember the last time he was in, which according to his medical record was about 4 years ago. Dr. Thompson's service is coded with an Office or Other Outpatient Services, New Patient.

1. Identify the defining trait to select Office or Other Outpatient Services

2. Identify the defining trait to select a new patient code

John is put in an exam room to wait for Dr. Thompson. While he waits, he starts getting the sensation he thinks is just bad heartburn. "Too much sausage at breakfast," he thinks. When Dr. Thompson comes in to see John, he asks John a number of questions about the heartburn, and John tells Dr. Thompson he's experiencing it currently. After a physical exam, Dr. Thompson decides to run a couple of tests on John right away in the clinic. Rather than heartburn, Dr. Thompson has determined John has been having cardiac chest pains that might be leading to a heart attack. Dr. Thompson leaves to give orders to his nurse for the tests.

While Dr. Thompson is gone, John gets sweaty, starts gasping for air, suddenly grabs his chest, and falls off the exam table. The nurse enters the room a few minutes later and finds John on the floor. She quickly hits the emergency button in the room and starts CPR on John. A receptionist dials 911 for a rescue squad, which transports John to the nearest emergency department. The emergency department physician, Dr. Singh, sees John immediately to assess his severe symptoms. Dr. Singh's service is coded with an Emergency Department Service.

3. Identify the defining trait to select an Emergency Department Service

Dr. Singh calls cardiology for a consult, which is performed by the cardiologist, Dr. Geld, who recommends a cardiac surgeon, Dr. Howard, be consulted to see if John is a candidate for emergent surgery. This is done, and Dr. Howard admits John to inpatient status in the hospital and performs a four-vessel bypass on John's heart.

Dr. Geld's service is coded as a Consultation.

CASE STUDY—cont'd

4. Identify the defining trait for a Consultation

Dr. Howard's service is coded as an Inpatient Hospital Service, Initial Service.

5. Identify the defining trait for an Inpatient Hospital Service

John has a complicated postoperative period but is finally ready to be discharged from the acute care hospital. However, John's wound hasn't healed properly and still needs close monitoring. The decision is made for him to stay at a local nursing home for a couple of weeks so he can receive daily wound care. Dr. Thompson admits John to a nursing home near his home so his wife can easily visit. After 2 weeks, John is released home to his wife.

Dr. Thompson's service is coded as a Nursing Facility Service.

6. Identify the defining trait for a Nursing Facility Service

Outpatient and Inpatient General Services

Chapter Outline

LEARNING OUTCOMES

On completion of this chapter, you will be able to:

1. Identify the seven E&M categories in this section.
2. Describe the defining trait of each category.
3. Classify each category as requiring "3 of 3" or "2 of 3" key components.
4. Recognize that each service category describes services provided in a particular physical location.

KEY TERMS

Consult 3 Rs	Nurse visit	Render
Emergency Department	One Rule	Report
Established patient	Outpatient	Request
Inpatient	Problem-oriented	Transfer of care
New patient	Referral	

Building on the Evaluation and Management (E&M) framework presented in Chapter 4, this chapter is the first of four that describe the E&M categories in detail. It introduces the first E&M categories listed in CPT; these are the majority of E&M categories used daily by most coders and include primary outpatient and inpatient service codes, observation status, same-day admit/discharge, consults, and emergency department services. When reporting these codes based on key components, it is imperative to identify whether two or three of the key components are required. However, some of the codes in this section are never reported based on key components, such as hospital discharge codes, and instead are reported based on time. Review in the CPT manual the E&M categories presented in this chapter.

Focus Questions

What are the three Rs of consult coding?

What is the deciding factor in using observation or inpatient service codes?

When a patient is admitted to the hospital from the clinic, how many E&M codes are reported?

What is the difference between an emergency department and an urgent care clinic?

■ OFFICE OR OTHER OUTPATIENT SERVICES (99201–99215)

Office or Other Outpatient Services is the first E&M category. It is the most commonly reported CPT code set because these are the primary codes used in physicians' offices. Both primary and specialty care physicians use these codes for every **problem-oriented** outpatient visit (as opposed to a preventive medicine visit). Of the defining traits listed in Chapter 4, this category has two defining traits—place of service and patient status.

⚠ KEY TERM

Problem-oriented—Visit in which a patient is treated for a presenting problem, as opposed to being seen for preventive care.

■ Examples of Office or Other Outpatient Services

- Patient presents to his family practitioner with flu-like symptoms.
- Patient seeks a second opinion regarding treatment options for atrial valve stenosis.
- Medical oncologist sees a patient in evaluation for chemotherapy.
- Ophthalmologist assesses visual changes in a patient with a 5-year history of glaucoma.
- Parent takes a child to an urgent care clinic status post fall from a bicycle.

The primary defining trait of these codes is place of service (Fig. 5-1). As discussed in Chapter 4, an **outpatient** place of service is any place of service not specifically defined as **inpatient** and is the more common of the two. Although these codes are usually used in the office setting, they are also reported in other outpatient locations. This may seem oversimplified, but coders commonly forget the title includes sites other than the physician office. Outpatient locations can include urgent care clinics, hospital-based outpatient departments, and observation status. Even though many of these physical locations have specific categories, Office or Other Outpatient Services is sometimes appropriate.

 CRITICAL THINKING

Why is an urgent care clinic more like a physician's office than an Emergency Department?
What nursing services could be reported with 99211?

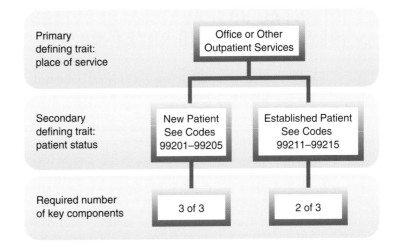

FIGURE 5-1 The Office or Other Outpatient Services category is divided into two subcategories, based on the secondary defining trait: patient status.

! KEY TERMS

Outpatient—A patient who is specifically not an inpatient in a hospital or nursing facility.
Inpatient—Specific admit status to a hospital or nursing facility.

The Office or Other Outpatient Services category is divided into two subcategories, based on the secondary defining trait of patient status (see Fig. 5-1). **New Patient** visits (patients not seen by the specialty practice group for more than 3 years) are reported with the five codes from 99201 through 99205 **3 of 3**. These codes increase in complexity from low to high in numeric order. Because a new patient typically requires a more comprehensive evaluation, this code series requires 3 of 3 key components to be documented at the minimum level listed.

Part 3 of this book includes detailed discussion of key components, the bolded portion of each code. At this point, it is important to understand that all codes in a series always have the same requirement: 2 of 3 or 3 of 3 key components must be met. Consider highlighting this difference in each code in the CPT manual, perhaps by using two highlighter colors.

The second subcategory is **Established Patient** visits, 99211 through 99215 **2 of 3**. These codes are used when a physician in the practice last saw a patient within 3 years of the date of service. Because these visits are usually less extensive, more focused, only 2 of 3 key component minimums are required. Similar to the codes for new patients, these five codes increase in complexity from low to high in numeric order.

! KEY TERMS

New Patient—A patient who has not received services from any physician in the specialty group practice within the last 3 years.
Established Patient—A patient who has received services from any physician in the specialty group practice within the past 3 years.

Code 99211 is unusual, as it does not necessarily require a physician see the patient. This is an exception to the face-to-face rule and is often referred to as a **nurse visit.** When an office nurse provides care incident to physician services that are not reported with a specific CPT code, such as 96372 for an intramuscular injection, report 99211.

! KEY TERM

Nurse visit—Visit in which the patient sees only a nurse, not a physician.

■ HOSPITAL OBSERVATION SERVICES (99217–99220 AND 99224–99226)

Place of service defines the Hospital Observation Services category (Fig. 5-2). Observation status in a hospital facility is necessary when reporting this code series. Best practice is to verify the patient's admit status with the hospital before coding physician services. Unlike the Office or Other Outpatient Services category, this is just a three-code series in addition to a discharge day code. Hospital admission evaluations are usually comprehensive, so 3 of 3 key component minimums are required. Determining the physical location of these services can be tricky, because hospitals frequently do not designate a unit for observation status patients but instead use rooms or beds on inpatient units, emergency departments, or extended-stay recovery rooms. The deciding factor for these codes is the admit codes, not the physical location.

There are three types of services reported for all admitted patients, whether observation or inpatient: (1) admit (initial) day services, (2) subsequent day services, and (3) discharge day services (see Fig. 5-2). Each of these applies to the calendar day and adheres to the **One Rule** (One physician, One code, One day). Initial Observation Care (99218–99220) **3 of 3** services report the care provided on the first calendar date of service. On the rare occasion that a patient in observation status is in the hospital for 3 or more days, the calendar dates between the admit date and the discharge date are reported with Subsequent Observation Care codes (99224–99226) **2 of 3** (see Fig. 5-2).

❗ KEY TERM

One Rule—The premise that a physician may report one E&M code per day for each patient seen. One physician, one code, one day.

Notice that the discharge services code, 99217, for observation status is first. This code does not require any key components, because the nature of discharge day services is different from admit or subsequent day services (see Fig. 5-2). Rather than being problem-oriented, the services focus on home care and necessary follow-up. If the admit and discharge services are performed on the same calendar

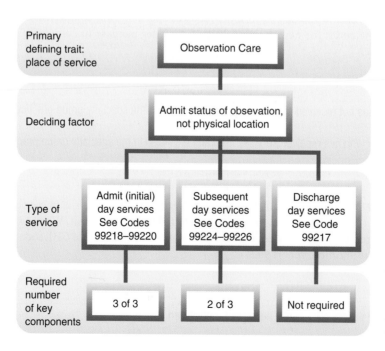

FIGURE 5-2 Place of service defines the Hospital Observation Services category. The three types of services reported for all admitted patients, whether observation or inpatient, are (1) admit (initial) day services, (2) subsequent day services, and (3) discharge day services.

date, report the services with a code from the Observation or Inpatient Care Services (Including Admission and Discharge Services) category, which is discussed later in this chapter.

 CRITICAL THINKING

When might a patient be admitted to observation status instead of inpatient status?

HOSPITAL INPATIENT SERVICES (99221–99223, 99231–99233, AND 99238–99239)

According to the CPT subsection guidelines, Hospital Inpatient Services, Initial Hospital Care (99221–99223) **3 of 3** , are used to report the E&M services of the admitting physician of record on the initial date of service for a patient admitted to an acute care facility. As with Hospital Observation Services, this category's defining trait is place of service, as described by the patient's admit status, and should be verified with the hospital facility before coding.

A code from this category may be reported only once per admission and only by the admitting physician. Payers that do not recognize consultation codes also allow each consulting physician to report a code from this category once per admission. The minimum requirements for these codes indicate that admission notes are expected to have a high level of documentation—at least a detailed history and exam.

Inpatient status is also the more important place of service, so if the same physician provides both outpatient and inpatient E&M services to the patient on the same date of service, report only the appropriate inpatient code (One Rule). However, documentation for all services is pooled to determine the appropriate level of service. A typical example is when admitting a patient directly from the physician office.

Subsequent Hospital Services (99231–99233) **2 of 3** describe E&M services provided on the days between the admit and discharge dates of service. The defining trait is place of service, inpatient. Some practices refer to these services as *rounding visits* or *floor visits*. Unlike the Initial Hospital Service subcategory, both admitting and consulting physicians report these codes for as many days as necessary. When a patient is in inpatient status, it may be necessary for the same physician to see a patient multiple times on the same date of service. Remember the One Rule. All documentation for services provided on the same date of service by the same physician is pooled to determine the appropriate level of service.

Services on the last day of inpatient status are reported from the subcategory Hospital Discharge Day Management (99238–99239). Similar to Observation discharge, this series does not utilize key components. Unlike Observation discharge, this series is reported based on documented time spent. If the documented time spent is 30 minutes or less, or if there is no documented time, report 99238. For services documented with time spent over 30 minutes, report 99239. The One Rule still applies, but for discharge services, the total time spent is added together from all notes on the final inpatient date of service. Discharge Day Management is the only appropriate code for the discharge date of service. If a subsequent hospital service is documented, and the patient is discharged later on the same date, that documentation is combined with any discharge notes to determine the appropriate level of service. If the admit and discharge service are performed on the same calendar date, report the services with a code from the Observation or Inpatient Care Services (Including Admission and Discharge Services) category.

OBSERVATION OR INPATIENT CARE SERVICES (INCLUDING ADMISSION AND DISCHARGE SERVICES) (99234–99236) **3 of 3**

The admit and discharge codes for both observation and inpatient status services are used on specific types of days during a patient's hospital stay. Those CPT guidelines, combined with the One Rule, require a third set of codes when the patient is admitted and discharged on the same date of service.

It is inappropriate to roll the discharge services into the admit services or vice versa. The requirements for the codes are also different. The defining trait for this category is type of service. This three-code series, more commonly referred to as Same Day Admit Discharge services, applies to both places of service—inpatient and outpatient—without regard to patient status. Pool all services provided on the date to determine the level of service. It is important to verify with the hospital facility that the admission and discharge occurred on the same calendar date. If the patient was admitted before midnight, then separate admit and discharge codes are used for each date of service.

 CRITICAL THINKING

Why are Same Day Admit and Discharge services codes defined by admitting and discharging the patient on the same date of service? Why are there not separate codes for this occurrence, based on place of service?

■ CONSULTATION SERVICES (99241–99245 AND 99251–99255) `3 of 3`

The type of service provided defines the Consultation Services category, which is divided into subcategories based on place of service—outpatient and inpatient (Fig. 5-3). Both series of codes have five levels of service. To determine whether an E&M service is a consultation, the **consult 3 Rs**—Request, Render, Report—must be documented. **Render** is simply documentation of the visit, with an assessment and plan associated with the request. **Report** is evidence that the consulting physician sent a written report to the requesting physician. The report may be completed in a variety of ways.

! KEY TERMS

Consult 3 Rs—Request, Render, Report.
Render—Documentation of a consultation visit.
Report—Evidence the consulting physician sent a written report to the requesting physician.

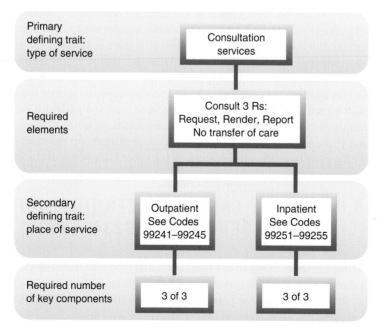

FIGURE 5-3 The type of service provided defines the Consultation Services category, which is divided into the subcategories of outpatient and inpatient. To determine whether an E&M service is a consultation, the consult 3 Rs must be documented.

▮ Examples of how to document the report portion of a consult

- The visit note is in letter form to the requesting physician.
- At the end of the visit note, the requesting physician is copied.
- A separate written letter exists in the medical record noting a copy of the visit note has been attached and sent to the requesting physician.
- The note is documented in a shared electronic medical record.

Request is a notation that a requestor has asked the consulting physician a question about a patient's condition and/or treatment options. Request can be more difficult to determine due to the varying nature of the language and intent of consultation services. A specific requesting physician must be noted, not a service or practice. Most medical providers, as well as other professionals, can request a consult, as long as the requestor can act on the information requested. In teaching physician hospitals, a resident physician may also be the requesting physician. There must also be some indication of the question asked, such as requesting that a definitive diagnosis be determined or the most effective treatment option for the patient be determined. The documentation required to prove a request was made can be rather difficult.

▯ KEY TERM

Request—Notation that a requestor has asked the consulting physician a question about a patient's condition and/or treatment options.

▮ Examples of adequate request documentation

- I was asked by Dr. Jones to see Ms. Patil today regarding treatment of her condition.
- Dr. Jones has sent Ms. Patil to see me today in consultation regarding treatment of her condition.
- Dear Dr. Jones, Thank you for asking me to see Ms. Patil regarding treatment of her condition.
- Ms. Patil is seen in clinic today at the request of Dr. Jones regarding treatment options for her condition.
- Patient: Ms. Patil. Requesting Physician: Dr. Jones. Request: Condition treatment options

▮ Examples of inadequate request documentation

- (No provider specified) I was asked by the medicine service to see Ms. Patil today regarding treatment of her condition.
- (Transfer of care instead of request) Dr. Jones has referred Ms. Patil to see me regarding treatment of her condition.
- (No evidence of a question) Dear Dr. Jones, I saw Ms. Patil today regarding treatment of her condition.
- (No requesting provider) Ms. Patil is seen in consultation today regarding treatment options for her condition.
- (Poorly worded template) Patient: Ms. Patil. Referring Physician: Dr. Jones. Concern: Condition treatment options

A **referral** is a recommendation to another medical provider without necessarily receiving any information in return. For coding documentation, a referral is not a consult; if the note states the patient was referred, then a consult has not occurred. For example, a patient who recently moved to a new city sees a local internist for an annual physical and, while there, asks the internist for the name of a nearby ophthalmologist. However, if the same patient complained of blurred vision, and the internist decides to have a specialist determine a diagnosis before treating the patient, a consult visit code would be appropriate.

Another requirement is that the visit not be a **transfer of care**. The requesting physician intends to continue treating the patient but needs more information on a specific issue. The consulting physician can initiate care and still report a consult but will not be responsible for the patient's entire treatment course. If the requesting physician sends the patient for a specific treatment or determines a diagnosis and refers the patient for the treatment the specialist concludes is needed but does not ask a question, then a transfer of care has occurred. An example is an Emergency Department physician sending a patient to a general surgeon for surgical treatment of cholelithiasis. The Emergency Department physician will not continue to care for the patient.

❗ KEY TERMS

Referral—Recommendation to another medical provider without necessarily receiving any information in return.

Transfer of care—Requesting physician sends a patient for a specific treatment or determines a diagnosis and refers the patient for whatever treatment the specialist concludes is needed but does not ask a question of the specialist.

When the consult 3 Rs are met, select a code based on the patient's place of service (see Fig. 5-3). Like Office or Other Outpatient Services, Outpatient Consultation Services (99241–99245) **3 of 3** are not limited to use in the office. These codes may be reported when rendering a consult in the Emergency Department, in observation status, in the hospital outpatient clinic, or in any other non-inpatient setting. If the consult 3 Rs are not met, then report an appropriate outpatient code.

Whether a patient is new or established does not affect the use of Outpatient Consultation Services. As long as the consult 3 Rs are met, a consult can be reported repeatedly. This may occur when a patient's condition is not yet severe enough to warrant treatment, so the requesting physician sends the patient to a consulting physician annually to determine disease progression. If the patient is seen for more than one visit in the course of the same consultation, report established patient visits after reporting the consult code once.

CRITICAL THINKING

What is the difference between the work performed by a physician when reporting a new outpatient visit versus an outpatient consultation?

For Inpatient Consultation Services (99251–99255) **3 of 3**, the consult 3 Rs still apply (see Fig. 5-3). Unlike an outpatient consult, an inpatient consult can be reported only once per admission per physician per consulting specialty, even if the requesting physician queries the consulting physician multiple times during the admission. All visits after the first visit are reported with Subsequent Hospital Services. If the patient is discharged and readmitted, the consulting physician may again report Inpatient Consultation Services once. If the consulting physician note in an inpatient setting does not include the consult 3 Rs, report a Subsequent Hospital Services code.

❋ Communicating With Medical Providers

The terms *consult* and *referral* can have different meanings for coders and physicians. From a medical standpoint, a physician might not make any distinction between a consult and a referral. Some specialty physicians consider all patients they treat to be consults because they do not see patients for primary concerns. Many physicians document that a patient was referred to them, when in coding terms the patient was sent for a consultation. When discussing consultation services from a coding perspective, do not discount these medical uses of the terms. Be clear that you are discussing consults and referrals in coding terms. Start the conversation by defining common terms, including *consult*, *referral*, *request*, and *transfer of care* so that everyone is speaking the same language. One way to differentiate a consult and a referral is that a consultation includes a communication loop between the requestor and the consultant. A referral does not have to include any communication between the requestor and the consultant.

■ EMERGENCY DEPARTMENT SERVICES (99281–99285) `3 of 3`

These five codes are reported only when services are rendered in an Emergency Department and are defined by place of service. An **Emergency Department** is accessible 24 hours a day, every day, and is physically attached to an acute care facility in the event a patient needs a higher level of care. Services rendered in an urgent care clinic, then, *are not* reported with Emergency Department Services but with Office or Other Outpatient Services. Every time a patient presents to the same Emergency Department, these services may be reported. New or established patient status does not apply to the Emergency Department, regardless of how many times the patient presents or the frequency of visits. Recall that any physician may report any CPT code. Therefore, use of the Emergency Department Services codes is not limited to designated emergency physicians.

! KEY TERM

Emergency Department—Accessible 24 hours a day, every day, and physically attached to an acute care facility in the event a patient needs a higher level of care.

CRITICAL THINKING

If it is difficult to remember, consider that Emergency Department Services includes the word *department* (of a hospital facility) and *Urgent Care* is short for *Urgent Care Clinic* (similar to a physician office). Why are urgent care and emergency services not reported with the same code set?

● ● ○ CHAPTER SUMMARY

- If reported based on key components, categories require either 2 of 3 or 3 of 3 key component minimums to be met.
- Office or Other Outpatient Services are reported for a variety of physical locations beyond the physician office.
- Verify the patient's admission status with the hospital medical record before selecting observation or inpatient codes.
- Apply the One Rule—each physician who sees a patient on any date of service may bill only one E&M code for that calendar date.
- The 3 Rs of consult coding are Request, Render, Report.

Chapter Review Exercises

1. Unless a place of service is specifically designated as inpatient, the place of service is _____.

2. Does code 99214, Office or Other Outpatient Services Established Patient level 4, require 2 of 3 or 3 of 3 key component minimums to be met?

3. Identify three physical locations where services from Office or Other Outpatient Services are reported.

4. How many E&M services may a physician report on a calendar date?

5. A patient's hospital admission status is either _____ or _____ and each has its own code categories.

6. How are services reported if a patient is admitted to inpatient status and discharged on the same day?

7. What if the patient in Question 6 is observation status?

8. The consult 3 Rs are:
   a. Refer, Request, Render
   b. Report, Render, Review
   c. Request, Render, Report
   d. Request, Request, Request

9. What are the defining characteristics of an Emergency Department?

10. The services in the categories in this chapter are _____, rather than preventive medicine services.

CASE STUDY

Anita Suarez is having right lower leg pain. Identify the service categories from which to report her care. Unless otherwise noted, assume that all services have been documented.

Ms. Suarez makes an appointment to see her internist, whom she last saw earlier this year for a sinus infection. The internist is concerned about Ms. Suarez's leg pain, as she also has type II diabetes and an increased risk for blood clotting. The internist decides he wants to get the opinion of a vascular surgeon before treating Ms. Suarez. The internist's office gives her the paperwork to set up an appointment.

Ms. Suarez sees the vascular surgeon about a week later and explains the pain she is having. The vascular surgeon thinks there is a blockage in the tibial artery, which requires surgery to correct. The vascular surgeon documents that the internist made the request and sends the internist a copy of the visit note with his opinion. The vascular surgeon is very concerned the clot blocking her tibial artery will become loose, which would be very dangerous. The vascular surgeon decides to admit Ms. Suarez as an inpatient first thing the day after the clinic visit to review further tests, start proper medication, and closely monitor the clot. The vascular surgeon sees Ms. Suarez on morning rounds. In the early evening, Ms. Suarez's pain suddenly increases, and the vascular surgeon sees her again. The vascular surgeon determines the pain was not due to the clot and continues her on her planned course.

While she is in the hospital, the vascular surgeon asks an endocrinologist to review how well her diabetes is controlled and if it is a contraindication for surgery. The endocrinologist sees Ms. Suarez the first day of her admission and documents the vascular surgeon's request and visit note in the shared record. While her condition does not rule out surgery, her blood sugar log shows some significant variation. The endocrinologist decides to visit Ms. Suarez daily to monitor this and proceeds to see her 3 additional days. The endocrinologist transfers care of her diabetes back to her internist upon discharge.

Ms. Suarez is in the hospital for a total of 5 days. The vascular surgeon sees her daily on morning rounds. On the fifth day, she is discharged from the hospital with instructions for rest, exercise, and revised medications. A week later, Ms. Suarez sees the vascular surgeon again to review how well she is doing. The pain has subsided and she is doing well on the medication. She also visits her internist that day, and he reviews how she is doing with a focus on better management of her diabetes. She notes she is enjoying the morning walks the vascular surgeon recommended and is trying to eat a better diet.

1. Internist visit

2. Vascular surgeon visit

3. Vascular surgeon hospital visit(s)

4. Endocrinologist hospital visit(s)

5. Vascular surgeon follow-up visit

6. Internist follow-up visit

6

Neonatal and Pediatric Specialty Services and Critical Care Services

Chapter Outline

LEARNING OUTCOMES

On completion of this chapter, you will be able to:

1. Identify the seven Emergency and Management (E&M) categories in this section.
2. Describe the defining trait of each category.
3. Name the type of service required to report each category.
4. Recognize whether a category has a time requirement.

KEY TERMS

Critical Care Services	Neonatologist	Obstetrician
Critically ill or injured patient	Newborn	Postpartum

The two types of services discussed in this chapter—neonatal and pediatric specialty services and Critical Care Services—are presented together because many of the definitions and requirements in the neonatal and pediatric specialty services section contain references to the Critical Care Services section. The primary difference between overlapping codes is the age of the patient. Most coders use the Critical Care Services codes, and only a small percentage of coders use the neonatal and pediatric specialty services categories. The latter coders are typically employed by neonatal specialty practice groups, children's hospital practice groups, and other similar specialty practices. These categories include newborn care, delivery/birthing room attendance and resuscitation services, pediatric critical care patient transport, inpatient neonatal and pediatric Critical Care Services, and continuing intensive care services. Unlike the categories in Chapter 5, these categories are reported based on the type of service delivered and, for some codes, the time spent treating the patient rather than on key components. As the E&M categories are presented in this chapter, also review the codes in the CPT manual.

Focus Questions

Why are initial hospital service codes not used to report normal newborn care?

Reporting Critical Care Services requires documentation of what two definitions?

In which places of service can Critical Care Services be reported?

How is neonatal critical care reported in an outpatient setting?

■ NEWBORN CARE SERVICES (99460–99463)

Newborn Care Services are reported only during the patient's initial care stay, from date of delivery to discharge. Normal **newborn** care, for a patient age 0 to 28 days, is not necessarily problem-oriented so it would be incorrect to report Hospital Inpatient Services. The newborn care services codes describe physician services for reviewing the mother's and newborn's history, a general newborn physical exam, and other typical newborn care. These patients may have minor problems but do not require intensive or critical care. Unlike most of the newborn and pediatric specialty codes discussed in this chapter, the newborn care services do not include any procedural services, so those should always be separately reported.

❗ KEY TERM

Newborn—Patient age 0 to 28 days.

 CRITICAL THINKING

If a newborn remains an inpatient from birth through more than 28 days, how would you report the care provided starting on day 29?

The defining trait of this category is type of service—care provided to a normal newborn. As noted in the CPT subsection guidelines, care of a normal newborn in either a hospital or birthing center is reported with 99460. Notice in the CPT manual that unlike the key component–based categories in Chapter 5, this category does not include levels of care but instead has different types of care defined by location and day of service. These codes also represent all care provided on the same date of service in keeping with the One Rule. When initial care is provided in any setting except a hospital or birthing center, such as in the patient's home, report code 99461. If normal newborn care is provided on additional days in a hospital, report 99462. When the newborn's admit (birth) and discharge services are on the same date, report 99463. There is not a specific code for normal newborn discharge on a different date than admission; in this case, report 99238 or 99239, Hospital Discharge Services.

 CRITICAL THINKING

Why is there not a code to report newborn discharge services in a non-hospital setting?

■ DELIVERY/BIRTHING ROOM ATTENDANCE AND RESUSCITATION SERVICES (99464–99465)

An **obstetrician** may ask a **neonatologist** to be present at a delivery because there is some identified risk to the baby that may require immediate care. When this occurs, the obstetrician should document the request. The neonatologist would then report *either* 99464 *or* 99465 for this service (Fig. 6-1). When the neonatologist is present for the birth and provides initial stabilization of the baby but does not

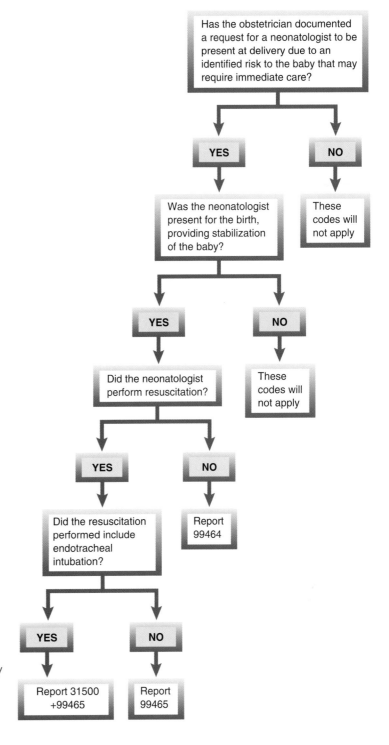

FIGURE 6-1 Defining Delivery/ Birthing Room Attendance and Resuscitation Services (99464 and 99465).

perform resuscitation, report 99464. If resuscitation is also required, report 99465. The work performed in these codes is acute and associated only with the period directly surrounding the birth. Therefore, code 99465 is not reported in addition to 99464. However, the delivery attendance codes may be reported in addition to normal newborn care codes, which represent more comprehensive services for the entire date of service.

If the standby request does not result in assisting the newborn in any way, the neonatologist may report Standby Service, 99360, for each 30 minutes spent. The physician may not be providing any other care or any other type of service during the standby time. Standby services may also occur during any request for a physician to be available, but 99360 is not reported if the time results in a procedure or other reportable service.

❗ KEY TERMS

Obstetrician—Physician specializing in pregnancy, birth, and maternal care.
Neonatologist—Physician specializing in newborn care and related diseases.

The codes in this category are defined by the type of service provided—attendance, initial stabilization, and perhaps resuscitation. Attendance does not just cover the physician in scrubs standing in the delivery room, but also includes reviewing necessary maternal and fetal historical information, reviewing lab and other diagnostic test results, and preparing for **postpartum** (after delivery) services. Initial stabilization may include drying and stimulating the baby, suctioning the baby's nose and mouth, performing an initial physical examination, providing accessory oxygen, and assessing Apgar scores.

Resuscitation services include assisted ventilation (positive pressure ventilation) and/or chest compressions (external cardiac massage). These codes do not include endotracheal intubation (31500). Code 99465 is reported when resuscitation is also performed. If the obstetrician requests and receives delivery attendance, but the neonatologist does not perform assisted ventilation and/or chest compressions, yet intubation is completed, report 99464 and 31500, not 99465. Review the Newborn Care Services guidelines in CPT (see Fig. 6-1).

 CRITICAL THINKING

Intubation can be part of helping a patient to breathe. When the neonatologist performs an intubation but does not perform assisted ventilation or chest compressions, why is 99465 not the correct code?

■ CRITICAL CARE SERVICES (99291–99292)

The most important concept for Critical Care Services is that the defining traits are patient status and type of service. To report Critical Care Services, the patient must be over 5 years and 364 days of age and must be critically ill or injured, which satisfies the patient status requirement. To meet the type of service requirement, Critical Care Services must be provided for at least 30 minutes (Fig. 6-2). These definitions are included in the extensive Critical Care Services subsection guidelines of CPT. Good comprehension of these definitions is crucial for proper use of the Critical Care Services codes. A **critically ill or injured patient** is one who has suffered significant impairment to at least one vital organ system or is at imminent risk of such impairment. The extent of the impairment is such that the patient's life may also be at risk. **Critical Care Services** include a physician's constant attention to one patient with a high level of effort to diagnose and treat the patient.

❗ KEY TERMS

Critically ill or injured patient—Patient who has suffered significant impairment to at least one vital organ system or is at imminent risk of such impairment.
Critical Care Services—A physician's constant attention to one patient with a high level of effort to diagnose and treat the patient.

✳ Communicating With Medical Providers

Physicians may be frustrated that third-party payers do not reimburse standby time (99360) because it is not considered medically necessary or because the physician is not providing active care. They then consider this to be a free service, which can be difficult when standby time becomes protracted. Consider that there are more ways to be reimbursed than by reporting services to a third-party payer. If the hospital requires standby time, it may have to reimburse the physician. This could be in the form of monthly invoicing, direct compensation, or program support. If it is the delivering physician's policy to request the standby time, a reimbursement agreement may be drawn up between the practices. Discuss with your physician and management whether they might pursue one of these avenues for proper reimbursement.

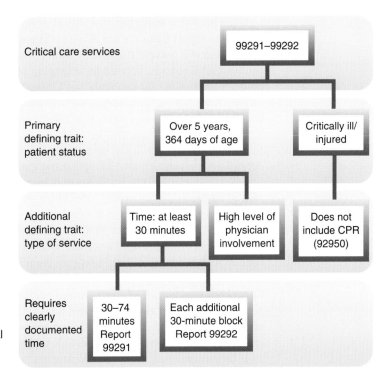

FIGURE 6-2 Defining Critical Care Services (99291 and 99292).

Critical Care Services will vary based on the patient's condition, but the nature of Critical Care Services is such that many decisions are made, many physiological studies are reviewed, and multiple procedures may be performed as part of a comprehensive care package; therefore, many study interpretations and procedures are included as part of Critical Care Services. However, if a procedure is performed that is not specifically included in Critical Care Services, it should be reported separately. One procedure not included in Critical Care Services is cardiopulmonary resuscitation (CPR), 92950. When a physician directs CPR, report it separately from Critical Care Services, and do not include the time spent directing CPR in the total critical care time (Table 6.1).

TABLE 6.1 Services Included in Reporting Critical Care Services

Description	CPT Code
Interpreting most physiological services, including:	
Cardiac output measurements	93561, 93562
Chest x-rays	71010, 71015, 71020
Pulse oximetry	94760, 94761, 94762
Blood gases	
Information stored in computers	
Reviewing vital signs	
Hematological studies	99090
Procedures:	
Gastric intubation	43752, 91105
Temporary transcutaneous pacing	92953
Ventilation management	94002–94004, 94660, 94662
Vascular access	36000, 36410, 36415, 36591, 36600

All other procedures performed may be separately reported and should not be included in the total critical care time spent. Refer to the CPT Critical Care Services section guidelines to verify the current list of included procedures.

If the patient is stable but critically ill or injured, there is an element of time involved in determining how to report Critical Care Services. The specific care provided needs to be provided at a specific time in order to prevent the patient from decompensating or to restabilize the patient. Services that can wait until rounds, or until an attending physician will usually be on the unit, or at some other point in the future, are probably not Critical Care Services as defined by CPT. Alternately, if the services documented appear to be Critical Care Services, but the patient is not critically ill or injured, the Critical Care Services codes may not be reported.

Critical Care Services may be provided in a wide variety of places of service. While they often occur in an emergency department or an intensive care unit, they may be provided anywhere the two definitions are met. A patient might suffer cardiac arrest in a physician's office and require Critical Care Services. Critical Care Services may be provided on a standard floor care unit, in an ambulatory area of a hospital, in an urgent care center, or even outside of a care facility.

The main Critical Care Services codes, 99291 and 99292, are time-based. The amount of time spent in Critical Care Services must be clearly documented to properly report. Code 99291 requires at least 30 minutes of critical care. If less than 30 minutes of care is provided, then another appropriate E&M code should be reported. Depending on the place of service, the code may be a Subsequent Hospital Care code or perhaps an Established Office or Other Outpatient Services code. Time spent in Critical Care Services includes time spent focused only on the critical patient. If time is spent overseeing multiple patients, no part of that time is counted toward Critical Care Services. If the services occur in an inpatient setting, all time spent focused on the patient at the bedside or on the floor/in the unit counts toward critical care time. This time might include reviewing records or speaking with other care providers.

If the patient is not able to participate in discussions about his or her own care, time spent with the patient's family or designated decision maker collecting information used to treat the patient or making decisions that affect the patient's care may be included in critical care time. That time must be bedside or on the patient's floor/unit so that the physician is immediately available to the patient.

Combine all time spent in Critical Care Services for a critically ill or injured patient, and report it once for the date of service. A patient might have more than one significant period in the day when Critical Care Services are required, or regular intervals of care might be required for the patient's condition. Time spent on the patient away from the patient's care area or time spent in the area but on other tasks may not be included in critical care time.

In addition, the time spent on separately reportable services is not included in critical care time. For example, if a Swan-Ganz catheter is placed, it is separately reported from Critical Care Services, so the time spent placing the catheter is not included.

Once 30 minutes of Critical Care Services is performed and documented, the critical care codes may be used. Code 99291 is reported for 30 to 74 minutes of Critical Care Services. The add-on code 99292 is used to report each additional block of 30 minutes (see Fig. 6-2). CPT includes an excellent table in the Critical Care Services guidelines to assist in properly coding these services. As long as the two definitions for Critical Care Services are met, these services may be reported on subsequent days. It is not unusual to see Critical Care Services reported for many days for trauma and burn patients, who require high-level care immediately postinjury.

✳ Communicating With Medical Providers

Physicians sometimes consider all services provided in an intensive care unit to be Critical Care Services or ICU services. They might also think that those services are all reported with Critical Care Services codes. Physicians believe care provided on a standard care unit and in an intensive care unit is discrete and so will often think the codes to report those services are similarly split into "floor" or "rounding" codes and "ICU" codes (Subsequent Hospital Services and Critical Care Services). It is important to ensure that everyone is using the same definitions for similar terms. Avoid telling physicians the services they are providing aren't critical care. From a medical perspective, they could be. However, reporting Critical Care Services codes requires specific definitions and thresholds of care. In conversations regarding Critical Care Services, keep clear the difference between what may be referred to as ICU services and the requirements for Critical Care Services codes.

The Critical Care Services guidelines also specifically note E&M services may be reported on the same date as Critical Care Services. Typically, the other service occurs first and then the patient becomes critical and critical care services are provided. A patient might be seen in the emergency room for a complete assessment and while waiting for further tests to be performed, or after admission, the patient's condition worsens. A patient might also be doing well on morning rounds and then require Critical Care Services later in the day. In this situation, the appropriate E&M code is reported with modifier -25, significant and separately identifiable evaluation and management service on the same day of the procedure or service, and the Critical Care Services are coded according to the total time spent on critical care.

A summary of requirements to report Critical Care Services is as follows:

■ The patient is critically ill or injured as defined by CPT.

■ The physician provides Critical Care Services as defined by CPT.

■ Critical Care Services may be provided in any place of service.

■ Reporting Critical Care Services requires at least 30 minutes of documented care.

■ Time spent must be bedside or on the patient's floor/unit.

■ Time may include time spent with decision makers if the patient is unable to make decisions.

■ Do not separately report included procedures.

■ Do not include time spent on separately reported services in the critical care total time.

■ Use the CPT Critical Care Services guidelines table for reporting with the add-on code.

■ CRITICAL CARE TRANSPORT (99288, 99466–99476, 99485–99486)

One of the places of service where Critical Care Services may occur is in transport. If a patient's condition requires that a physician attend to the patient during transport, the Critical Care Services definitions are met, and at least 30 minutes of Critical Care Services are documented, then the main Critical Care Services codes, 99291–99292, may be reported. However, if the physician is not in face-to-face contact with the patient, the Critical Care Services codes do not apply. Instead, if the physician directs the patient's emergency care or advanced life support remotely via two-way communication while the patient is being transported, and the patient is over 24 months of age, then 99288, Physician Direction of Emergency Medical Systems (EMS) Emergency Care, Advanced Life Support, is reported. For patients 24 months of age or younger, report the service based on the total time spent directing care with the code range 99485–99486.

If the patient is 24 months of age or younger, and the patient's condition requires that a physician accompany the patient in transport, and the critical care definitions are met, report codes 99466–99467, Pediatric Critical Care Patient Transport. As with the main Critical Care Services codes, report 99466 for at least 30 to 74 minutes of services provided, and report add-on code 99467 for each additional 30-minute time block. The physician's reportable time spans beyond the time spent while physically in transport. It starts when the physician takes responsibility for the patient at the referring facility and ends when the physician transfers care to a physician at the receiving facility.

Unlike the main Critical Care Services codes, the Pediatric Critical Care Patient Transport time includes time spent face-to-face with the patient. Pediatric Critical Care Patient Transport includes all of the services encompassed in the main Critical Care Services and all of the serevices included in Inpatient Neonatal and Pediatric Critical Care. Tables 6.1 and 6.2 list these procedures. Any additional procedures performed by the physician, but not by any of the transport personnel, may also be reported. Remember not to include time spent on those procedures in the total time for the Pediatric Critical Care Patient Transport.

 CRITICAL THINKING

What defining trait is missing to report Pediatric Critical Care Patient Transport with the codes 99468 through 99476?

TABLE 6.2 Services Included in Reporting Inpatient Neonatal and Pediatric Critical Care

Description	CPT Code, if Applicable
Invasive and noninvasive vital sign monitoring	
All vascular access, including:	36000, 36140, 36620, 36510, 36555, 36400, 36405, 36406, 36420, 36600
Airway and ventilation management	31500, 94002–94004, 94375, 94610, 94660
Monitoring and interpreting blood gases or oxygen saturation	94760–94762
Blood transfusions	36430, 36440
Oral or nasogastric tube placement	43752
Suprapubic bladder aspiration	51100
Bladder catheterization	51701, 51702
Lumbar puncture	62270

All other procedures performed may be separately reported and should not be included in the total critical care time spent. Refer to the CPT Critical Care Services section guidelines to verify the current list of included procedures.

■ INPATIENT NEONATAL AND PEDIATRIC CRITICAL CARE SERVICES (99468–99476)

The Inpatient Neonatal and Pediatric Critical Care Services codes represent all of the physician work performed to care for a critically ill or injured neonate or child. These services have separate codes from the main Critical Care Services codes because they usually on the date of service involve assessing the patient many times during the day, interacting with parents or guardians and other care providers, and providing many services throughout the day. The definitions of a critically ill or injured patient and of Critical Care Services are the same for the Inpatient Neonate and Pediatric Critical Care Services as they are for the main Critical Care Services category. These codes are always reported once per calendar date and by one physician. All of the procedures listed in Table 6.1 are also included in the Inpatient Neonatal and Pediatric Critical Care Services. The procedures in Table 6.2 are included in these codes.

Because these services occur throughout the day and include time spent on many services, they are not reported based on time; rather, one code is reported per date of service, regardless of the time spent with the patient. Instead, the codes are reported based on age: 28 days of age or younger (99468–99469), 29 days through 24 months (99471–99472), and 2 to 5 years 364 days (99475–99476) (Fig. 6-3). There is a code in each age range for the initial date of service (99468, 99471, 99475) and a code for subsequent dates (99469, 99472, 99476). Remember that Critical Care Services provided to children 6 years old and over are reported with 99291–99292.

The Inpatient Neonate and Pediatric Critical Care codes have a few rules about reporting. If a physician provides Delivery/Birthing Room Attendance and Resuscitation Services, 99464–99465, on the same date as 99468, Initial Inpatient Neonatal Critical Care, both codes may be reported. Also, any procedures performed in the delivery room may be separately reported, even if they would otherwise be included in the Neonatal Critical Care Services, as they were provided before Critical Care Services began. Good documentation that these procedures were necessary at the time they were provided is essential. If the procedure is performed incidentally in the delivery room but is actually part of the Critical Care Services, it should not be separately reported.

As noted in the subsection guidelines for these codes, another unusual reporting situation occurs if a neonatal or pediatric patient is transported between two facilities and the patient receives Critical Care Services at both of those facilities on the same date of service. If the physicians providing the services at each facility are from different practice groups, the physician at the sending facility should report 99291–99292 for Critical Care Services, and the physician at the receiving facility should report an appropriate Inpatient Neonatal and Pediatric Critical Care Services code (99468, 99471, or 99475). If the physicians are in the same practice group, the physician who provides a majority of the services that day would report the appropriate Inpatient Neonatal and Pediatric Critical Care code based on patient age and day of care.

Notice that these critical care codes are specifically for inpatient services, unlike the main Critical Care Services codes. When a neonate or child receives Critical Care Services in an outpatient setting,

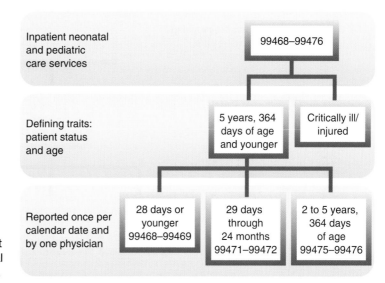

FIGURE 6-3 Defining Inpatient Neonatal and Pediatric Critical Care Services (99468–99476).

and the definitions and time requirements are met, report the main Critical Care Services codes 99291–99292. These services most likely will occur in the Emergency Department or when the patient is in observation status, but they may also occur in the many other outpatient places of service.

■ INTENSIVE CARE SERVICES

When a neonate is no longer critically ill but continues to require extensive daily monitoring and assessment, such as monitoring cardiac and respiratory function, heat maintenance, or other vital life support, Intensive Care Services may be reported. These codes include the same procedures as outlined for Critical Care Services and Inpatient Neonatal and Pediatric Critical Care Services but do not require the critical care definitions to be met. These patients are often still in an intensive care unit but are more generally stable than patients requiring critical care. For neonates 28 days of age or younger who require intensive care services, report 99477 for all care provided on the initial date of service, similar to 99468 (Fig. 6-4).

The subsequent Intensive Care Services codes are assigned according to the neonate's weight. For neonates weighing under 1500 grams, report 99478. Intensive Care Services for neonates weighing 1500 to 2500 grams are reported with 99479. Report 99480 for neonates weighing 2501 to 5000 grams. Care provided to neonates over 5000 grams and all non-Critical Care Services provided to infants and children over 28 days of age are reported with Subsequent Hospital Care (99231–99233) services (see Fig. 6-4).

●●○ CHAPTER SUMMARY

- ■ Neonatal and Pediatric Specialty Services and Critical Care Services are defined by the type of service provided and patient status.
- ■ Newborn care services are provided only to the newborn patient during the first care admission.
- ■ Delivery/Birthing Room Attendance and Resuscitation Services are defined by whether resuscitation was required.
- ■ Critical Care Services require that the patient be critically ill or injured and received critical care services for at least 30 minutes per date of service.
- ■ Critical Care Transport includes only physician face-to-face time with the patient.
- ■ If the physician is directing care remotely, report Physician Direction of Emergency Services.
- ■ If the patient is 24 months of age or younger, report Pediatric Critical Care Patient Transport.
- ■ Report Inpatient Neonatal and Pediatric Critical Care Services based on the patient's age and whether the date of service is initial or subsequent.
- ■ Use Intensive Care Services for neonates with low birth weight who require intensive monitoring but who aren't critically ill.
- ■ Infants and children over 5000 grams who require intensive or other care have services reported with Subsequent Hospital Care codes.

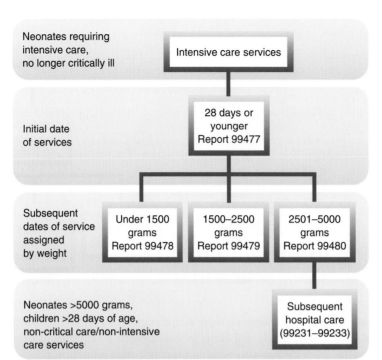

FIGURE 6-4 Defining Neonatal Intensive Care Services.

Chapter Review Exercises

1. What is the minimum time that must be documented to report the main Critical Care Services codes?

2. Which neonate Intensive Care Services code should be assigned for a baby weighing 1500 grams?

3. How old must an infant be to report codes 99471 and 99472?

4. What are the two definitions that must be met to report Critical Care Services?

5. True or false: Codes 99291 and 99292 should be reported only when the patient is being treated in a critical care unit or emergency department.

6. What code is reported for care provided to a newborn on the delivery date in the patient's home?

7. If the neonate is born in a hospital, what code is used to report discharge services on admission day 3?

8. How many minutes of critical care must be documented to report 99291 and 99292×1?

9. If a physician provides 45 minutes of Critical Care Services to an 18-month-old patient during transport, should the reported code be 99291, 99466, 99485, or 99288?

10. An infant is discharged from the hospital the day after delivery. However, the infant develops jaundice and is readmitted when 5 days old. Should the Newborn Care Services codes be used for the readmission? Why or why not?

CASE STUDY

Carole has been on bed rest in inpatient status at Grace Hospital for a week in an attempt to prevent premature labor. Unfortunately, at 30 weeks gestation, Carole enters active labor. Because the infant will be born prematurely and likely need assistance immediately postpartum, Carole's obstetrician asks a neonatologist to stand by at the delivery. The neonatologist arrives along with a nurse trained to care for premature newborns. At birth, the obstetrician hands over baby boy, Jacob, to the neonatologist who immediately begins to stabilize Jacob by drying him and suctioning out his nose and mouth. Jacob's 1 minute Apgar score is 5, with absent breathing and a blue complexion. The neonatologist determines Jacob will need significant assistance breathing and performs an endotracheal intubation. The nurse begins positive pressure ventilation through the endotracheal tube. At 5 minutes, Jacob's Apgar is 8 and he's considered stable enough to transfer to the neonatal intensive care unit (NICU). Jacob is weighed and measured in the NICU, coming in at 1,319 grams and 39 cm long, which is about average for his gestational age.

Jacob's critical state required that he remain in the NICU for some time. The neonatologist provided critical care services for 7 days total, including the delivery date of service.

Identify the neonatologist code(s), if applicable, for each date of service:
Day 1
Day 2
Day 3
Day 4
Day 5
Day 6
Day 7

On Day 8, Jacob remained critical and it was determined he should be transferred to the local children's hospital for more specialized care. His weight in the NICU that day was 1,372 grams. Early that morning, he was transported to the children's hospital. Because of Jacob's critical state, the neonatologist accompanied him on the trip. The neonatologist assumed responsibility for Jacob at 7:15 a.m. and transferred care to the neonatal pulmonologist at the children's hospital at 8:45 a.m. The neonatal pulmonologist provided critical care services to Jacob for the remainder of the day.

1. Identify the neonatologist code(s) at Grace Hospital, if applicable.
2. Identify the neonatologist code(s) in transport, if applicable.
3. Identify the neonatal pulmonologist code(s), if applicable.

CASE STUDY—cont'd

Jacob remained critically ill, and the neonatologist provided critical care services through Day 15. On Day 16, Jacob was doing much better, and while he wasn't yet ready to leave the NICU, he was no longer critical. The neonatologist continued to see Jacob multiple times a day, providing intensive care services through Day 25. Jacob's weight was charted daily on Table 6.3:

TABLE 6.3   Jacob's Weight Chart

Age (Days)	Weight (Grams)
1	1319
2	1328
3	1340
4	1352
5	1360
6	1365
7	1368
8	1372
9	1368
10	1373
11	1377
12	1390
13	1402
14	1419
15	1444
16	1464
17	1487
18	1512
19	1547
20	1576
21	1609
22	1655
23	1693
24	1745
25	1789

Identify the neonatologist code(s) (or code category), if applicable, for each date of service:
Day 9
Day 10
Day 11
Day 12
Day 13
Day 14
Day 15
Day 16
Day 17
Day 18
Day 19

Continued

CASE STUDY—cont'd

Day 20
Day 21
Day 22
Day 23
Day 24
Day 25

While in the NICU, Jacob continued to improve under the neonatologist's care. On Day 45, he weighed 2,485 grams. This was his last day of intensive care in the NICU. On Day 53, he was sent home with his mother with instructions for proper feeding to continue his weight gain and ways to avoid respiratory infections. A nurse would visit him to monitor his home progress.

Identify the neonatologist code(s) (or code category), if applicable, for each date of service:
Day 45
Day 53

Patient Home Services

Chapter Outline

LEARNING OUTCOMES

On completion of this chapter, you will be able to:

1. Identify the patient residence place of service.
2. Describe the defining trait of each category in this chapter.
3. Differentiate between face-to-face services and care plan oversight.
4. Classify each category as either a time-based service or one that requires "3 of 3" or "2 of 3" key component minimums to be met.

KEY TERMS

Assisted living	Care plan oversight	Home

The defining trait for services in this chapter is place of service. The services reported with categories in this chapter are all performed in or affect care in the patient's home or place of residence. Patients can reside in a variety of settings, such as nursing homes, boarding homes, or assisted living facilities. The categories covering these services include Nursing Facility Services; Domiciliary, Rest Home (e.g., Boarding Home or Assisted Living Facility), or Custodial Care Services; Home Care Plan Oversight Services; and Home Services. As with the categories in Chapter 5, these categories are reported based on the key components (except for care plan oversight).

Focus Questions

Is a nursing facility an inpatient or outpatient place of service?

Is the patient's private home an inpatient or outpatient place of service?

Why is care plan oversight by a physician necessary?

What category should be used for psychiatric residential treatment center services?

■ NURSING FACILITY SERVICES (99304–99318)

As described in Chapter 4, **nursing facilities** are inpatient places of service because patients receive both room and board and skilled nursing care. Nursing facility admissions frequently occur on the same date of service as other evaluation and management (E&M) services. When a patient is discharged from an acute care setting and admitted to a nursing facility on the same date of service, both the appropriate discharge code and the appropriate initial nursing facility care code may be reported. The admitting physician may also perform some of the work of an initial nursing facility care visit in another place of service. When that occurs, all portions of the initial nursing facility care service are reported with the initial nursing facility care subcategory, in accordance with the One Rule. For example, the physician might initiate a patient's admission history and physical in the office and complete the Resident Assessment Instrument (RAI) in the nursing facility. Both of those services are part of the initial nursing facility care (Fig. 7-1).

❗ KEY TERM

Nursing facilities—Facilities that provide care for patients still in need of monitored nursing care but who no longer require care for acute illness or injury.

CPT divides the Nursing Facility Services category into Initial Nursing Facility Care and Subsequent Nursing Facility Care. Initial Nursing Facility Care (99304–99306) **3 of 3** is reported only once per nursing facility admission by the admitting physician on the initial date of service (see Fig. 7-1). Similar to Initial Hospital Care (99221–99223), there are three levels of service in this category that represent comprehensive services to review the patient's history and status, to determine a care plan for the patient's stay that considers all of the patient's current diagnoses and comorbidities, and to write admitting orders. Because a nursing facility admission is sometimes of some length, this visit will also include planning for the patient's room setting and family considerations.

Subsequent Nursing Facility Care (99307–99310) **2 of 3** is similar to Subsequent Hospital Care (99231–99233). All providers treating the patient in a nursing facility setting may use these codes to report services (see Fig. 7-1). Services reported with Subsequent Nursing Facility Care codes include

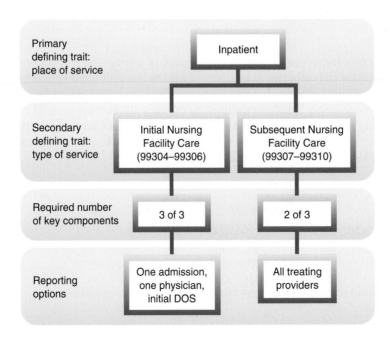

FIGURE 7-1 Nursing facility inpatient services.

both initial treatment of a patient for a new problem and the interval review of a patient for existing problems by a treating physician. This category includes four levels of service, one more than similar categories. The fourth code (99310) describes a level of service that is typically more urgent than the other levels and is used when the patient is unstable or has developed a significant new problem requiring immediate attention.

Because patients often stay in nursing facilities for extended periods, they must be evaluated annually regardless of condition to determine updated care plans. This visit may be mandated by a regulating body. When a physician provides this non–problem-oriented service, report Other Nursing Facility Services (99318) **3 of 3** . This visit typically involves completing required forms and providing the patient with a thorough visit including a review of records and tests performed since the patient was last seen as well as a comprehensive examination.

Finally, as with Hospital Inpatient Services, there is a specific category for Nursing Facility Discharge Services (99315–99316). Services provided on the discharge date might include reviewing instructions for home care, exercises, updated prescriptions, and upcoming physician appointments. If the documented time spent is 30 minutes or less, or if there is no documented time, report 99315. Services documented with time spent over 30 minutes are reported with 99316. All of the time the physician spends with the patient performing discharge services is combined and reported with one Nursing Facility Discharge Services code.

DOMICILIARY, REST HOME (E.G., BOARDING HOME), OR CUSTODIAL CARE SERVICES (99324–99337)

Place of service defines the Domiciliary, Rest Home (e.g. Boarding Home), or Custodial Care Services category. These outpatient facilities are similar to nursing facilities in that they provide room and board and personal assistance services, but they do not include a nursing service component. This category

✳ Communicating With Medical Providers

E&M services coding can often seem subjective and hard to relate to the services rendered. While they cannot be used alone to choose services, there are many tools in CPT that can assist you in discussing E&M service categories and codes with physicians.

1. Become familiar with all of the category guidelines and definitions. Highlight and underline important information, and make pertinent notes next to the guidelines. Take your CPT book with you to physician meetings so you have your notes and bookmarks that are familiar to you.

2. There is a rationale behind why each category has differing numbers of levels of service. The last paragraph of each code usually describes the typical conditions that result in the code being reported. An example is those paragraphs for the Subsequent Nursing Facility Care category (99307–99310):
     99307—Usually, the patient is stable, recovering, or improving.
     99308—Usually, the patient is responding inadequately to therapy or has developed a minor complication.
     99309—Usually, the patient has developed a significant complication or a significant new problem.
     99310—The patient may be unstable or may have developed a significant new problem requiring immediate physician attention.
     Share this information with the physician to facilitate a discussion of what code best represents the service required and whether the elements of that service were performed. That last paragraph also includes the typical time spent on a service, which can be a good guide as well.

3. Remember, Appendix C includes clinical examples developed by a wide variety of physician specialty organizations for every E&M category. Highlight those for your specialty, and use them in discussions with physicians. Make sure to communicate that they were developed by the physician's own specialty. This can help guide you both to the appropriate category or code for the service provided.

also includes physician services performed in **assisted living facilities.** The category is subdivided into New Patients (99324–99328) `3 of 3` and Established Patients (99334–99337) `2 of 3` (Fig. 7-2). This subdivision refers to the patient's status—whether new or established with the physician, not with the facility.

！ KEY TERM

Assisted living facilities—Similar to nursing facilities in that they provide room and board and personal assistance services, but they do not include a nursing service component.

Services performed in assisted living communities can be difficult to correctly report. Assisted living communities often include multiple levels of care where a resident may begin living in a completely independent apartment. The resident might then move into an assisted living setting that includes personal assistance with daily care. If the patient has an episode requiring nursing care or a chronic illness that requires long-term nursing care, the patient might then move into a nursing facility portion of the same community. If the patient's status is unclear, contact the facility to verify before selecting a category.

■ DOMICILIARY, REST HOME (E.G., ASSISTED LIVING FACILITY), OR HOME CARE PLAN OVERSIGHT SERVICES (99339–99340)

Some patients may not require nursing services but still require significant oversight of their care plan by a physician. These codes are time-based services and are defined by the type of service provided. Face-to-face time with the physician is not required, and the services are typically performed without the patient present. A variety of services can be included in the total time used to select a code. Time spent reviewing patient status reports, laboratory and other diagnostic study results, and adjusting medical therapy may be included. A significant portion of the time spent might be in communication with other health care professionals, family members, surrogate decision makers, and caregivers regarding assessment of the patient and decisions regarding care.

This is also the first category presented so far that covers services for more than one date of service. The total time spent in **care plan oversight** per calendar month is reported with a single code. Clear time documentation is key to reporting these services properly. If the total time spent is 15–29 minutes, report 99339. If the total time is 30 minutes or more, report 99340. If less than 15 minutes of care plan

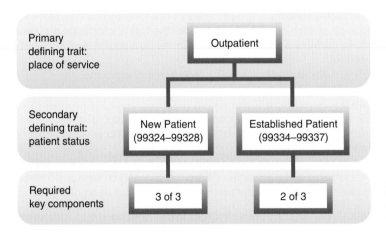

FIGURE 7-2 Outpatient domiciliary, rest home, or custodial care services.

oversight services are provided in a calendar month, the service is not reported. Note that 99340 is not an add-on code, so report either 99339 or 99340, but not both codes.

KEY TERM

Care plan oversight—Management of all patient services without face-to-face services; may include a variety of services including time spent reviewing patient status reports, laboratory and other diagnostic study results, adjusting medical therapy, and communication with other health care professionals, family members, surrogate decision makers, and caregivers regarding assessment of the patient and decisions regarding care.

These codes are used only for care plan oversight of patients living in one of the defined places of service. If the patient is enrolled with a home health agency, in hospice, or residing in a nursing facility, this category should not be selected (see Care Plan Oversight Services in Chapter 8).

■ HOME SERVICES (99341–99350)

Physician services rendered in the patient's home are reported with this category. The patient's **home** is a private residence with no coordinated care services. The home place of service defines the category, which is further subdivided into New Patient (99341–99345) **3 of 3** and Established Patient (99347–99350) **2 of 3** . The patient's status as new or established is determined by the patient's history with the physician and does not refer to whether the patient is new or established to the place of service or whether the physician has previously seen the patient at home (Fig. 7-3).

KEY TERMS

Home—A private residence with no coordinated care services.

 CRITICAL THINKING

Why are there different categories for nursing facility, assisted living facility, and home services?

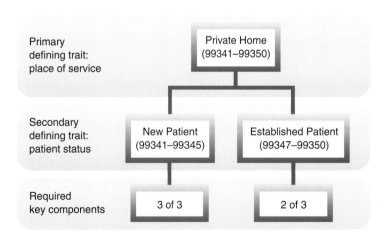

FIGURE 7-3 Home services. *Patient status defined by patient's history with the physician, not place of service.

CHAPTER SUMMARY

- Categories in this chapter are largely defined by the patient's living arrangement.
- From most intensive care to least, those places are: nursing facilities, assisted living facilities, and home.
- Nursing facilities provide long-term skilled nursing services.
- Assisted living provides personal care assistance.
- Home is the patient's private residence where no organized care is provided.
- Care plan oversight services do not require the patient's presence.

Chapter Review Exercises

1. When a patient is discharged from an acute care (hospital) facility and admitted to a nursing facility on the same date of service, what, if any, category should be selected?

2. If a physician renders services to a patient living in an assisted living community, but in an independent private apartment, what category should be reported?

3. How are 10 minutes of home care plan oversight reported?

4. Is the patient's home an inpatient or outpatient place of service?

5. The order and use of Nursing Facility Services categories are similar to Hospital Inpatient Services categories. The order and use of Domiciliary, Rest Home (e.g. Boarding Home), or Custodial Care Services and Home Services are similar to Office and Other Outpatient Services. Why?

6. A physician renders discharge services to a patient in a nursing facility for 20 minutes. If the service can be reported, should it be reported as 99239 or 99315?

7. A patient has recently moved into a rest home and the patient's current internist visits the patient there for a scheduled visit. To select the correct category, is it more important that the patient is new to the rest home or established to the physician?

8. What three questions should be asked before selecting a category and subcategory for services rendered to a patient living in a blended care assisted living community?

9. A cardiologist is asked to consult on a patient. The cardiologist sees the patient at the nursing facility where the patient resides and communicates an opinion back to the patient's internist. Should the cardiologist report a code from the Consultations category or from the Nursing Facility Services category?

10. In question 9, is the correct subcategory Inpatient Consultation, Office or Other Outpatient Consultation, Initial Nursing Facility Care, or Subsequent Nursing Facility Care?

CASE STUDIES

Assign the appropriate category. Note if no code should be reported.

1. A 78-year-old female patient with an 8-year history of Parkinson disease is ready to be discharged from an acute care hospital post-fall that caused a pelvic fracture. The internist sees the patient bedside to discuss discharge.

2. The patient's current diagnoses also include insulin-controlled type II diabetes mellitus. The patient's Parkinson disease has advanced to a stage where she is no longer able to ambulate independently and requires assistance for basic hygiene and daily care. Her 80-year-old spouse feels unable to provide this care safely following the fall. The patient's internist determines that the patient also requires close monitoring of her diabetes and Parkinson disease sequelae to a degree that it is decided to admit the patient directly from the hospital to a local nursing facility on the same date of service. The internist sees the patient in the nursing home later that same day.

3. The internist sees the patient again a week later to assess how she is adapting to the nursing facility and whether she is continuing to heal from her fall.

4. A couple of months into her stay, the patient complains of reduced vision. Her internist stops by to see her and assesses her vision. The internist decides to ask an ophthalmologist for an opinion.

5. The ophthalmologist sees the patient the next time he is at the nursing facility. He determines the patient has lid ptosis and recommends blepharoplasty to correct the condition. The ophthalmologist dictates a letter to the internist regarding his opinion.

6. Two weeks later, the patient leaves the nursing facility to have the blepharoplasty performed as an outpatient at the local hospital.

7. She returns to the nursing home later that evening.

8. Two days later, the ophthalmologist stops by to check on how the patient is healing and confirms she is doing well.

9. The patient continues to be stable in the nursing facility. A year after her admission, the internist performs an annual nursing facility assessment for the patient. It is noted at that visit that the patient is once again experiencing vision problems. The internist asks the ophthalmologist to see the patient again.

10. The ophthalmologist stops by to see the patient and determines her cataracts have advanced to a stage that they are causing vision impairment and should be removed. He writes a letter to the internist noting this finding.

CASE STUDIES—cont'd

11. After cataract surgery, the patient regains some ability to care for herself. The patient continues to do well and is eventually deemed ready for discharge. The internist sees her on the date of discharge for an hour to discuss her move, treatment plan, and medications.

12. The patient moves into an assisted living community on the same date of service.

13. A week later, the internist checks on the patient in her new assisted living community where she does not receive nursing care but does receive personal assistance care.

14. Because of the patient's complicated medical history, the internist continues to monitor her care plan and make adjustments as necessary.

Other Services

Chapter Outline

LEARNING OUTCOMES

On completion of this chapter, you will be able to:

1. Identify the nine Evaluation and Management (E&M) categories in this chapter.
2. Describe the defining trait of each category.
3. Name the type of service required to report each category.
4. Recognize whether a category has a time requirement.

KEY TERMS

Add-on codes	Non–face-to-face	Structured screening
Face-to-face	Preventive medicine	Unlisted service

This chapter describes the final E&M categories. These categories do not have any common trait except that they all describe unusual and often very specific care situations. The defining trait for these services is primarily type of service. None of these services employ key components, but instead they have specific guidelines by category. The categories include prolonged services, case management services, care plan oversight services, preventive medicine services, non–face-to-face physician services, special E&M services, complex chronic care coordination, transitional care management (TCM), and other services.

Focus Questions

When may prolonged services codes be applied?

In what instance are a preventive medicine service and an office visit billed on the same date of service?

What time constraints apply to telephone services?

What is the difference between case management and care plan oversight?

Do the discharge day services count toward TCM requirements?

■ PROLONGED PHYSICIAN SERVICE WITH DIRECT (FACE-TO-FACE) PATIENT CONTACT (99354–99357)

Occasionally a provider may spend an extended amount of time with a patient that is significantly longer than the usual time spent in a particular service. When that occurs, **face-to-face** prolonged services may be reported. As face-to-face prolonged services do not occur without another service being provided, these services are reported with **add-on codes.** Prolonged services are reported in addition to any E&M service that includes a typical time spent and at any level in a series of codes (Fig. 8-1).

The first set of prolonged services codes is for face-to-face services. In the outpatient setting, this means time spent by the provider directly with the patient. No time spent away from the patient may be counted. However, if the care is provided in the inpatient setting, time spent on the patient's unit or floor, such as at the nursing station working on the patient's case, may also be considered. All time spent working with the patient on the date of service may be combined when reporting prolonged services. The time does not need to be continuous (see Fig. 8-1).

At least 30 minutes beyond the primary service's typical time are required to report prolonged services. In the outpatient setting, this time is reported with 99354. This code reports 1 hour of service. The second outpatient code 99355 is for each additional 30 minutes. Note that both 99354 and 99355 are add-on codes. Code 99355 is never used without 99354. Code 99354 represents the first hour, and 99355 represents each additional 30 minutes in excess of that first hour. Similar to critical care (99291–99292), at least 15 minutes must be spent to report 99355. Table 8.1 describes the time cut-off for each code. If the patient is an inpatient, codes 99356 and 99357 are used in a similar fashion (see Fig. 8-1).

⚠ KEY TERMS

Add-on codes—CPT codes that are only reported in addition to another CPT code.

 CRITICAL THINKING

Why can face-to-face prolonged services codes not be added to services that do not include a typical time?

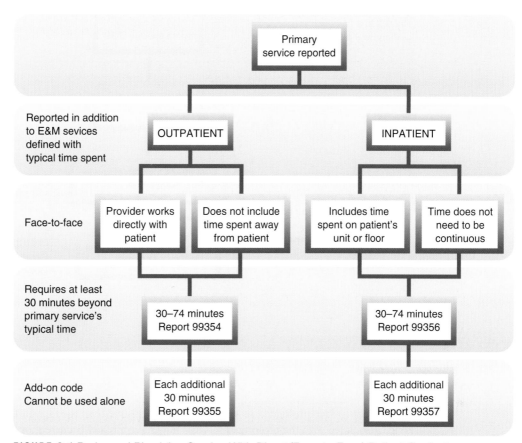

FIGURE 8-1 Prolonged Physician Service With Direct (Face-to-Face) Patient Contact.

TABLE 8.1 Prolonged Services Reporting by Time

Time Spent in Prolonged Services	Coding
1–29 minutes	Not separately reported
30–60 minutes	+99354
61–74 minutes (1 hour and less than 15 minutes)	+99354
75-104 minutes (1 hour 15 minutes–1 hour 44 minutes)	+99354, +99355
105–134 minutes (1 hour 45 minutes–2 hours 14 minutes)	+99354, +99355x2

■ PROLONGED PHYSICIAN SERVICE WITHOUT DIRECT (FACE-TO-FACE) PATIENT CONTACT (99358–99359)

These codes are reported when significant **non–face-to-face** time is spent on a patient's care but does not include non–face-to-face time for which specific codes exist, such as case management or medical team conferences. While there must be a primary service to which these services relate, non–face-to-face prolonged services may be reported on a separate date of service. Because of this, the first code, 99358, for the first hour of service is not an add-on code. It may be reported independently. The second code in the pair, 99359, for each additional 30 minutes, is an add-on and must be reported in addition to 99358. The time spent on a service does not need to have been continuous; the total time is reported (Fig. 8-2). Reporting codes 99358 and 99359 works the same as the codes listed in Table 8.1.

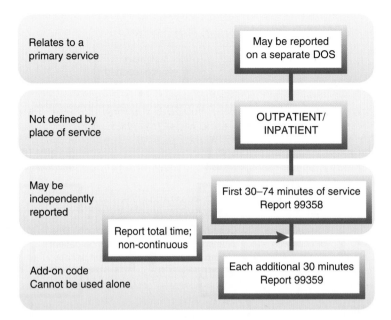

FIGURE 8-2 Prolonged Physician Service Without Direct (Face-to-Face) Patient Contact.

! **KEY TERMS**

Non–face-to-face—Work that is not in the physical presence of the patient.

Non–face-to-face prolonged services are less constrained than the face-to-face codes. The primary service associated with the prolonged services may have already occurred, or it may occur in the near future. The services may be reported in addition to E&M services that do not have a typical time. There is no distinction made for the patient's place of service. Other non–face-to-face services may serve as the primary service, with prolonged service codes used after the primary service's time maximum is reached.

Prolonged Services can seem intimidating. Following the rules in Table 8.1 is a good foundation for coding these services. The most important concept to remember is that the usual time spent on a service is not included in calculating Prolonged Services units.

 CRITICAL THINKING

Why is there more flexibility in reporting non–face-to-face prolonged services?

CASE MANAGEMENT SERVICES (99363–99368)

Case Management Services encompass services provided by a physician who has a treatment relationship with a patient and who is also overseeing the patient's comprehensive care, as defined in the specific types of case management services. The patient is not present when the physician renders these services. Case Management Services include Anticoagulant Management and Medical Team Conferences.

ANTICOAGULANT MANAGEMENT (99363–99364)

Physicians provide Anticoagulant Management for patients on warfarin therapy. Warfarin is a drug that works to thin the blood and prevent coagulation. It is also known by brand names such as Coumadin. These patients require regular monitoring to ensure the patient maintains therapeutic drug levels. Anticoagulant Management includes ordering and interpreting the patient's International

TABLE 8.1 Reporting Prolonged Services

Remember these rules when reporting prolonged services:

1. Prolonged services may be reported with any level of service within a series of E&M codes.
2. Choose face-to-face or non–face-to-face codes as they apply.
3. Prolonged services total time does not need to be continuous on the date of service.
4. The second add-on code in a pair is always used with the pair's first add-on code, never alone.
5. Reporting a unit of the second add-on code requires at least 15 minutes of prolonged services beyond the last unit of time.

Face-to-Face Prolonged Services
6. Select outpatient or inpatient codes based on the patient's place of service.
7. These services may only be reported with E&M codes that include a typical time.
8. Time included when calculating prolonged services does not include the primary service's typical time.

Non–Face-to-Face Prolonged Services
9. Services may occur on a date of service different from the primary service.
10. Make no distinction between outpatient and inpatient services.
    Must relate in some way to a primary service.

Normalized Ratio (INR) lab value, drug management, and communicating lab results and medication adjustments to the patient.

Anticoagulant Management represents services provided on multiple dates of service. These codes represent all related services provided within a continuous 90-day period. The physician must provide services for at least 60 days to report the service. To report 99363, the physician must complete at least eight INR measurements in 60–90 days. After the first reporting period, the physician must complete at least three INR measurements for every 60–90 day period. If the physician provides a significant, separately identifiable E&M service within the reporting period, it is reported with modifier -25. (Fig. 8-3)

Should the patient become an inpatient, reporting of anticoagulant management ceases, and the reporting period is reset at discharge using 99364. Reporting ceases even if the provider initiates anticoagulant management in the inpatient place of service and regardless of the length of the inpatient

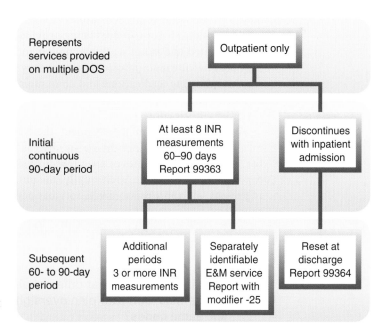

FIGURE 8-3 Anticoagulant Management.

stay. Because of this, do not report 99363 and 99364 with inpatient and observation stay codes, critical care codes, or other services that already include anticoagulant management.

■ MEDICAL TEAM CONFERENCES (99366–99368)

Medical Team Conferences are reported when at least three health care providers meet to discuss a patient's care. The providers must be from different specialties, and only one provider per specialty may report any one medical team conference. All providers who are going to report this service must have treated the patient independently within the 60 days before the conference. Each provider reporting medical team conferences must document his and her own participation in the conference and any decisions he or she as a part of the review. Physicians may not report contractually required conferences, such as tumor board.

Providers who report medical team conferences must actively participate in the conference and be present for the entire time they report. Time reported for medical team conferences does not include time spent record keeping or generating reports, only the active review time for the patient. The providers must spend at least 30 minutes reviewing the patient's care to report these services.

When the patient is present for the medical team conference, physicians report an office visit or other appropriate E&M service with time as the key factor. Only non-physician providers may report 99366. This code is reported when the patient is present and includes any conference time period of 30 minutes or more. If the patient is not present, physicians report 99367 and non-physician providers report 99368. Notice that a blend of codes may be reported for the same medical team conference, based on the types of providers participating in the conference.

CRITICAL THINKING

Why are different codes reported for (1) physicians and non-physician providers and (2) for conference with the patient present and not present?

■ CARE PLAN OVERSIGHT SERVICES (99374–99380)

Physicians provide Care Plan Oversight Services when a patient requires oversight of care provided in the home by a home health agency (99374–99375), in hospice care (99377–99378), or in a skilled nursing facility (99379–99380). The oversight must be more than the low intensity oversight that will occur as part of other E&M services. In essence, the physician acts as a manager for all of the patient's care, which requires regular monitoring. Care Plan Oversight Services include physician supervision of the patient who requires complex and multidisciplinary care. The physician will typically be reviewing multiple care services being provided to the patient in the same period to ensure the care is coordinated and is not working counter to any other care provider concurrently. The physician may be reviewing multiple care reports as they are rendered, monitoring laboratory and radiological studies, adjusting medications and communication as necessary with care givers and the patient's decision makers. CPT includes extensive guidelines for this category of codes, which should be reviewed in their entirety.

As with anticoagulant management, these codes report services provided over a period of time—a calendar month—rather than a specific date of service. The first code of each pair is reported for the first 15–29 minutes of oversight provided in a calendar month. The second code is reported for 30 minutes or more. Additionally, the patient is never present for these services. If the patient is present, an appropriate E&M services code, such as a home visit or nursing facility visit, is reported.

CRITICAL THINKING

Identify the activity that differentiates anticoagulant management, medical team conference, and care plan oversight. Why are these services not all reported with the same codes?

■ PREVENTIVE MEDICINE SERVICES (99381–99387 AND 99391–99397)

Providers render **Preventive Medicine Services** when the patient does not present with a specific complaint (Fig. 8-4). *Annual physicals, sports physicals, school physicals,* and *well-child checks* are some of the other names for preventive medicine. An important concept to remember is that the comprehensive preventive service is not the same as a comprehensive history or exam required to report high level office visits or other basic E&M services. The comprehensive preventive medicine service includes an age- and gender-appropriate history and exam and applicable risk factor screening and reduction counseling. Many specialty societies have published recommended preventive services for all life stages.

! KEY TERMS

Preventive Medicine Services—Physician service to prevent disease; patient presents without specific complaint.

■ Examples of age- and sex-specific preventive medicine services

- A 73-year-old woman presents for an annual physical. Discussion includes osteoporosis prevention, screening for arthritis and dementia, and counseling regarding staying active with chair exercises. Blood is drawn to check glucose and cholesterol.
- A 55-year-old male presents for an annual physical. The physician encourages the patient to have a colonoscopy performed in the next few months. The exam includes a prostate exam, and labs are drawn to check the patient's PSA. They discuss a heart healthy lifestyle, and the physician screens the patient for any symptoms of heart disease.
- A 6-month-old infant presents with his father for a well-child check. The baby's height and weight are measured to ensure proper growth. The nurse practitioner discusses various developmental milestones with the father and whether there is any concern for those milestones not yet met. Because the baby has started scooting and will soon crawl, they discuss baby proofing, such as covering wall outlets. Using a properly installed car seat at all times is emphasized.

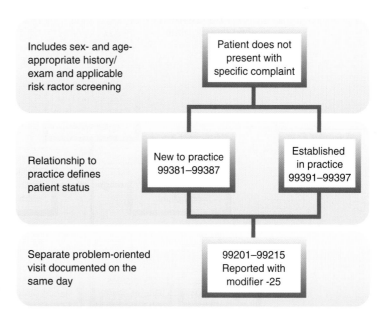

FIGURE 8-4 Preventive Medicine Services.

Codes 99381–99387 are reported for patients new to the practice—not for the patient's first preventive care visit. Codes 99391–99397 are reported for patients established in the practice. See Table 8.2 for a description of which code to use at what age. Although the care provided should be gender-specific when appropriate, the preventive service codes are not gender-specific. Table 8.2 identifies Preventive Medicine Services by patient age and whether the patient is new or established to the practice.

If a patient presents for a preventive medicine service but also has a significant complaint, or if a significant problem is discovered during the visit and additional work is required that would not usually be performed as part of the preventive medicine service, a separate problem-oriented office visit (99201–99215) may be reported with modifier -25 (see Fig. 8-4). The office visit should be well documented to support reporting the service.

■ COUNSELING RISK FACTOR REDUCTION AND BEHAVIOR CHANGE INTERVENTION (99401–99429)

Codes in this section are similar to Preventive Medicine Services but describe services based more on discussion and counseling than physical exam. They are reported for services provided to a patient who presents without a specific complaint. As with Preventive Medicine Services, a significant and separately identifiable E&M service may be reported on the same date of service with modifier -25 (Fig. 8-5).

All of the services in this section are time-based. Preventive Medicine, Individual Counseling (99401–99404) describes time spent with a patient, one-on-one, discussing risk factor reduction. The discussion will vary based on the patient's age, gender, personal habits, and family history. Unlike many of the E&M codes, Preventive Medicine, Individual Counseling, is not billed by unit. Instead, the four codes in the series describe a total approximate time spent with the patient. These codes are not add-on codes; only one code is reported for the correct time spent. For example, if about 30 minutes are spent counseling the

TABLE 8.2 Preventive Medicine Services

Age	New Patient	Established Patient
Under 1 year (0–11 months)	99381	99391
1–4 years (1 year–3 years 11 months)	99382	99392
5–11 years	99383	99393
12–17 years	99384	99394
18–39 years	99385	99395
40–64 years	99386	99396
65 years or older	99387	99397

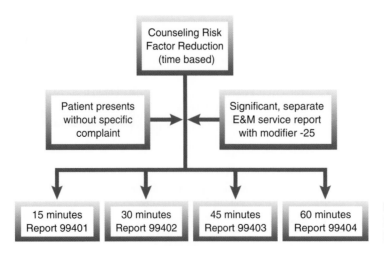

FIGURE 8-5 Counseling Risk Factor Reduction and Behavior Change Intervention.

patient, 99402 is reported alone. (Code 99401 is used to report 15 minutes, 99403 to report 45 minutes, and 99404 to report counseling lasing 60 minutes) (see Fig. 8-5).

Behavior Change Interventions, Individual (99406–99409) describe counseling services for specific habits (Fig. 8-6). Codes 99406–99407 Smoking and Tobacco Use Cessation Counseling Visits, are reported for specifically discussing tobacco cessation with a patient, one-on-one. Note that 99406 requires at least 3 minutes spent counseling the patient, up to 10 minutes. Code 99407 describes any amount of time counseling the patient over 10 minutes. Codes 99408–99409 Alcohol and/or substance (other than tobacco) abuse structured screening (e.g. AUDIT, DAST) and structured brief intervention (SBI) services are reported for abuse of other substances than tobacco. The codes require that a **structured screening** process be completed (see Fig. 8-6). Code 99408 is reported for counseling lasting 15–30 minutes, and 99409 is reported for counseling more than 30 minutes.

❗ KEY TERMS

Structured screening—A preconceived screening method to assess a patient condition.

Codes 99408–99409 require some type of structured screening be completed as part of the intervention. The AUDIT and DAST are just two examples of a wide variety of structured screenings that may be utilized when reporting these codes. Other examples include MAST, CAGE, CRAFFT, T-ACE, and TWEAK. A care provider administers the screening by asking a series of questions or the patient completes a questionnaire to assist the provider and patient in assessing the patient's level of substance use or abuse and what risks are associated with that use.

Preventive Medicine, Group Counseling (99411–99412) codes are reported for group counseling regarding risk factor reduction. Report 99411 when the counseling session lasts approximately 30 minutes and 99412 for approximately 60 minutes. These codes are similar to Preventive Medicine,

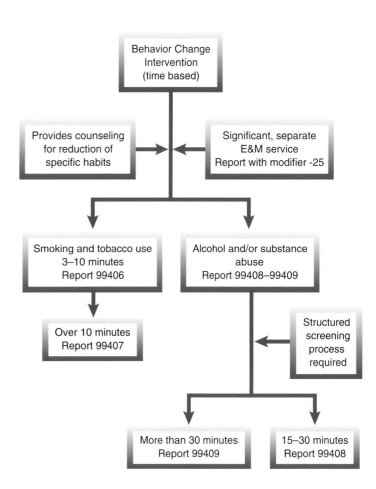

FIGURE 8-6 Behavior Change Interventions, Individual.

Individual Counseling, but are used in a group setting. The code is reported once per session per participant.

■ OTHER PREVENTIVE MEDICINE SERVICES (99420–99429)

There are just two codes in this section. The first, 99420, Administration and Interpretation of Health Risk Assessment Instrument (e.g., health hazard appraisal), is reported for administering or reviewing any applicable assessment, except alcohol or substance abuse. The assessment might concern the patient's work environment, the patient's home environment, a behavioral assessment such as screening for domestic violence, or possible exposure to a harmful substance or disease.

The second code is 99429, Unlisted Preventive Medicine Service. In the event a Preventive Medicine Service is rendered that does not have an exact code, this code may be reported. More often, the payer may direct the practice to use this code for a certain service.

■ NON–FACE-TO-FACE PHYSICIAN SERVICES (99441–99444)

Non–face-to-face physician services require that a face-to-face service by the same provider have not occurred within the last 7 days. However, the patient must be established with the practice. Even though the physician may not respond immediately, the patient must initiate these services. Only physicians report these codes (Fig. 8-7). Qualified non-physician providers report codes from CPT Medicine (98966–98969).

Telephone Services (99441–99443) also may not result in a face-to-face service in the next 24 hours or at the next available urgent appointment time. The time associated with the service includes only time spent in medical discussion. Telephone Services may be reported only once every 7 days. As well, a telephone service may not be reported within 7 days of a reported on-line service (see Fig. 8-7). The physician must spend at least 5 minutes in medical discussion with the patient or patient's guardian by telephone to report Telephone Services. Code 99441 is used to report discussions lasting 5–10 minutes. Code 99442 reflects 11–20 minutes of medical discussion, and 99443 reflects 21–30 minutes of medical discussion.

The physician may conduct an On-Line Medical Evaluation, 99444, in any format, including e-mail and chat (see Fig. 8-7). However, the communication must be stored permanently to report 99444. This code is not time-based and is reported for all on-line services provided during any 7-day period by the same physician. Additionally, any other services related to the on-line service are included in reporting this code, including calling in prescriptions and ordering tests.

■ SPECIAL E&M SERVICES (99450–99456)

Special E&M Services are reported specifically for establishing the patient's baseline health information for life or disability insurance. The place of service may be the office or any other outpatient place of service. These services can be reported for new and established patients. These codes do not include

Non–face-to-face physician's services	Telephone services	On-line medical evaluation
• No face-to-face within last 7 days	• No face-to-face service within next 24 hours	• Any format including e-mail and chat
• Patient status established with practice	• Includes only time spent in medical discussion	• Communication must be permanently stored
• Codes reported only by physician	• Must spend at least 5 minutes in medical discussion	• Not time-based
		• Includes other related services (prescriptions, test orders)

FIGURE 8-7 Non–Face-to-Face Physician Services.

any active evaluation and management of any current conditions or those discovered in the course of the service. A significant and separately identifiable E&M service may be reported on the same date of service with modifier -25. See Figure 8-7.

Code 99450, Basic Life and/or Disability Examination, should include a number of services, including measuring the patient's height, weight, and vital signs. Typically, the service also includes taking a medical history as required by the insurance issuer, collecting blood, urine, and/or stool samples for analysis, and completing any required documents.

Work-Related or Medical Disability Evaluation Services (99455–99456) assess the patient's ability to work and/or level of disability with regard to eligibility for disability benefits and services. Report 99455 when the patient's treating provider completes the service, and 99456 for any other provider. The activities included in this service are all related to the patient's disabling condition: completing a medical history, completing a physical exam, making a diagnosis, assessing the degree of disability, developing a treatment plan, and completing any necessary documentation.

 CRITICAL THINKING

Why are disability evaluation services not simply reported with Office Visit or Preventive Medicine Services codes? How are they different?

■ COMPLEX CHRONIC CARE COORDINATION (99487–99489)

Complex Chronic Care Coordination (CCCC) is reported for services provided to patients with one or more chronic conditions and that require coordination of multiple services. These patients have a high likelihood of additional medical or psychiatric and behavioral co-morbidities. Patients requiring CCCC frequently also lack strong social support of healthy living and lack access to care either due to distance or access to transportation.

Similar to Care Management Services, CCCC represents all outpatient care provided within a calendar month rather than on a specific day. The service is provided by the patient's primary care physician and includes care for all medical conditions; any psychosocial needs such as maintaining housing, scheduling transportation, and setting appointments; and activities of daily living. Many of services included in CCCC will be provided by support staff in the clinic environment. When there is not a clinic or home visit during a calendar month in which CCCC occurred, 99487 is reported. If there is one clinic or home visit during the month, the first hour of CCCC, including time spent during the visit, is reported with 99488. Each additional 30 minutes spent in CCCC during that calendar month is reported with 99489. CCCC should not be reported until after the calendar month so that the total time expended can be totaled. Any additional clinic or home visits during the month are reported separately with the appropriate E&M Category (Fig. 8-8).

■ TRANSITIONAL CARE MANAGEMENT SERVICES (99495–99496)

The goal of Transitional Care Management Services (TCM) is to avoid readmission within the first 30 days following discharge from an inpatient acute care hospital, partial hospital, observation status, or skilled nursing facility. Patients requiring TCM often have significant psychosocial and daily living needs that increase the likelihood of readmission. One code from the series is reported by the patient's established primary care physician during the 30-day care period in which day 1 is the date of discharge (Fig. 8-9).

Regardless whether the physician who will report TCM also discharged the patient, following discharge, the reporting physician must make meaningful contact—not just scheduling the face-to-face service—with the patient within 2 business days of discharge. Initial contact may be face-to-face, by telephone, or electronic. If contact cannot be made within the first 2 business days, two or more separate attempts to contact the patient must be documented in the medical record.

TCM includes one face-to-face visit with the reporting physician. If the patient's medical complexity is moderate, the visit must occur within 14 days of discharge, and TCM is reported with 99495.

Complex Chronic Care Coordination 99487–99489

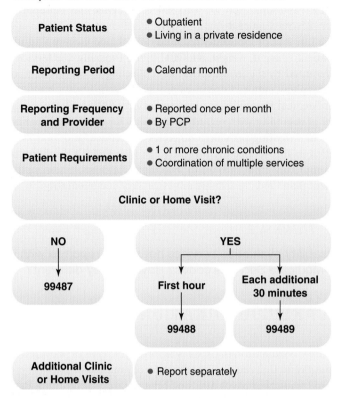

FIGURE 8-8 Complex Chronic Care Coordination Services.

Transitional Care Management Services 99495–99496

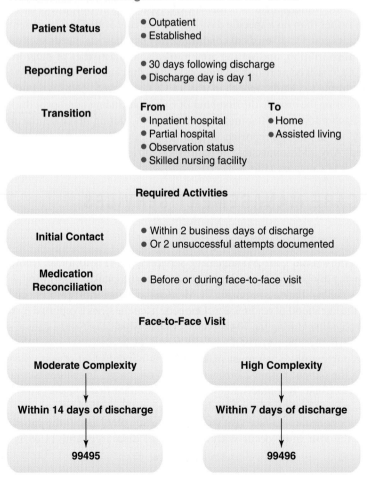

FIGURE 8-9 Transitional Care Management Services.

For highly complex patients, as defined by CPT Medical Decision Making, the face-to-face visit must occur within 7 days, and TCM is reported with 99496. If the face-to-face visit for highly complex patients occurs 8–14 days from discharge, the service may still be reported, but with 99495. The reporting physician must also complete a medication reconciliation for the patient sometime between discharge and the end of the face-to-face visit. As with CCCC, any additional face-to-face visits may be reported separately with the appropriate E&M category.

TCM and CCCC both include most services provided during the reporting period by the reporting physician and clinic staff. See Figure 8-10 for a complete list of included services.

■ OTHER SERVICES

There is just one code in Other Services, 99499, Unlisted Evaluation and Management Service. In the event an E&M service is rendered that does not have an exact code within the E&M section, this code may be reported. More often, the payer may direct the practice to use this code for a certain service.

 CRITICAL THINKING

Can you think of an E&M service that was not described in the CPT E&M chapter that would be reported with 99499?

CCCC and TCM Services include:

- Care Plan Oversight Services
- Prolonged Services Without Direct Patient Contact
- Anticoagulant Management
- Medical Team Conferences
- Education and Training
- Telephone Services
- ESRD Services
- Online Medical Evaluation
- Special Reports Preparation
- Data Analysis
- Medication Therapy Management
- TCM (when reporting CCCC)
- CCCC (when reporting TCM)

FIGURE 8-10 CCC and TCM Service Inclusions.

 Communicating With Medical Providers

The services in this chapter are distinct and usually require a specific service to be completed, which actually makes reporting the codes straightforward. However, different payers do not cover many of these services. This can be troubling to a physician who finds the service to be medically necessary and vital to the patient's good health. It is important to understand which payers with which your practice contracts cover what services. Do not fall into the trap of assuming if Medicare does not cover a service that it is never covered. For example, whereas Medicare does not cover telephone services, a local HMO may reimburse these services because the HMO has found it increases patient satisfaction and reduces emergency department utilization. The practice should keep a grid of these services to ensure proper billing.

Engage your physicians and other billing providers in the process of understanding which payers cover these services. They may want to set up a process for patients in certain plans to communicate with them via e-mail. As well, this is a good time to discuss when patients may need to pay out-of-pocket for services versus third party payment. The key is not to inform the providers that they can or cannot provide a service. Of course, they are better equipped to determine what services are medically necessary. The discussion should focus on how best to be reimbursed for those services once they are provided.

●●● SUMMARY

- Prolonged services can be reported with any other E&M code that includes a typical time.
- Case management services are reported for anticoagulant management or medical team conferences, which have service specific requirements.
- Three or more health care professionals who have treated the patient within the last 60 days must actively participate in order to report a medical team conference.
- Care plan oversight services codes represent all oversight services provided during a calendar month and are reported based on the patient's place of service.
- The patient's age and relationship to the practice define Preventive Medicine Services.
- Telephone and on-line services cannot be separately reported when the physician reported an E&M service in the previous 7 days.

Chapter Review Exercises

1. Why are face-to-face prolonged services codes add-on codes?

2. Once the E&M service's typical time is spent providing the service, how many minutes must be spent to report a face-to-face prolonged service?

3. What time frame is represented by codes 99363 and 99364?

4. How many INRs must the physician complete to report 99364?

5. When a non-physician care provider participates in a non–face-to-face team conference, what code is reported?

6. How many physicians may report care plan oversight services during 1 calendar month?

7. Select the preventive medicine code to report for services provided to a 37-year-old female patient who was last seen by the practice 4 years ago.

8. What code is reported for spending 75 minutes assessing a patient's level of cocaine use and counseling the patient regarding ending this habit?

9. If a physician sees a patient on Monday, what is the next day 99442 may be reported for a patient-initiated telephone call including 15 minutes of medical discussion?

10. Assign a TCM code for the services provided to a moderately complex patient who is seen in the clinic 5 days following discharge. (Other TCM requirements are met.)

CASE STUDY

Assign the appropriate category. Note if no code should be reported.

1. Martin is a long-time patient of his gerontologist, Dr. Johnson. He presents in July for his annual check-up. Dr. Johnson discusses Martin's overall feeling of health with him, his social habits, and his relationship with his wife. He then completes a comprehensive physical exam. Dr. Johnson lets Martin get dressed and returns to discuss a variety of risk factors with Martin, including heart disease risk factors, his use of a seatbelt in automobiles, and maintaining good physical health through exercise. They discuss Martin's high blood pressure in some detail, as Dr. Johnson is concerned that Martin is not keeping it well controlled with diet.

2. Two weeks later, Martin remembers he wanted to ask Dr. Johnson about whether he would benefit from taking a certain supplement that is said to lower blood pressure. He calls the office and leaves a message. Dr. Johnson calls him back later that evening, and they spend about 10 minutes discussing the pros and cons of the supplement and whether a prescription medication might be more effective.

3. Dr. Johnson calls Martin a few days later to discuss a new study he just read concerning the high blood pressure medication they had discussed. They agree Martin should come in to the office soon for a blood pressure check and to make some decisions about treating his high blood pressure.

4. Martin returns to the office a few weeks later and sees Dr. Johnson. Dr. Johnson completes and documents services reported with 99214. Dr. Johnson also engages in a lengthy discussion of how to treat high blood pressure, including discussing various studies Dr. Johnson has read, information Martin found on the Internet, and the dangers of having uncontrolled high blood pressure. In total, Dr. Johnson and Martin spend 60 minutes together. By the end of the visit, Martin is still unsure how he wants to treat his high blood pressure. Dr. Johnson strongly counsels him to begin medication soon.

5. Before Martin came in for that visit, Dr. Johnson spent about an hour reviewing Martin's medical records. He created a chart of Martin's blood pressure readings over time to review with Martin. He also gathered some medical study information to share with Martin at the visit.

6. Unfortunately, Martin did not start treating his high blood pressure, and he suffers a stroke. The stroke is significant enough that Martin suffers some late effects, including slurred speech and right-sided weakness. Once he is well enough, Martin moves from the hospital to an inpatient rehabilitation facility. In order to return as much of Martin's function as possible, his care providers meet regularly to discuss his progress. On the first Tuesday of each month for 1 hour, Dr. Johnson meets with Martin's speech pathologist, occupational therapist, and neurologist to review how Martin is doing and what changes in care might improve his condition.

CASE STUDY—cont'd

7. Martin continues to improve and eventually moves home. The day after discharge, Dr. Johnson's nurse calls Martin at home to see whether he was settling in and taking his medications. They discussed his activity level and warning signs to watch for complications. Dr. Johnson visits Martin at home 10 days after discharge and determines he is progressing well. Martin is able to maintain his exercise program, and his wife is monitoring his medications, which Dr. Johnson reconciles while he is there. Dr. Johnson's staff continues to work with Martin throughout the 30 days following discharge to prevent readmission, which strategy is successful.

8. After 6 months, Martin's therapists determine his physical disabilities have improved as much as they are going to. Dr. Johnson sees Martin to evaluate him for disability benefits. He completes Martin's medical history and a complete exam of his ability to move his right side. Dr. Johnson determines Martin will always need to use a walker or wheelchair for mobility and is unable to grasp anything smaller than a soup can with his dominant right hand. Dr. Johnson completes the forms Martin needs to submit with his request for benefits.

Evaluation and Management Services—Levels and Components

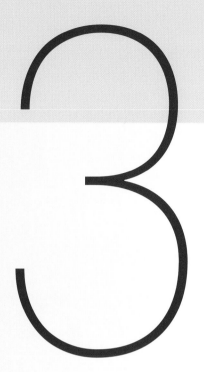

9

Evaluation and Management Service Level Selection

Chapter Outline

I. Soap Note Format

II. E&M Components

III. Coding Methods—Key Component-Based Codes

IV. Coding Methods—Code Specific Service

LEARNING OUTCOMES

On completion of this chapter, you will be able to:

1. Identify the seven components of an Evaluation and Management (E&M) Service.
2. Identify the two coding methods.
3. Describe the structure of a key component-based code description.
4. Differentiate which codes require 2 or 3 of the key component minimums to be met.
5. Select correct codes when the service is not component-based.

KEY TERMS

Assessment	Key components	Objective
Contributory Components	Medical Decision Making	Plan
Coordination of Care	Medical necessity	SOAP Note
Counseling	Nature of Presenting	Subjective
Examination	Problem	Time
History		

E&M code descriptions include abundant guidance describing the code and the service it represents. Understanding not only the key components of a service but also the contributing components is essential to selecting the correct E&M code. It is important to identify whether a component-based code requires 2 or 3 of the key component minimums to be met. Many of the E&M service codes are component-based, but there are notable exceptions that are reported according to specific directions for the service. For those services, time spent providing the service is often critical to selecting the correct code.

Focus Questions

What are the 3 key components?

What are the 3 contributing components?

What is the 7th component?

How many of the key component minimums must be met in order to report a component based code?

If a code is not selected based on key component documentation, what element is most often used to determine a code?

■ SOAP NOTE FORMAT

Physicians are often taught in medical school to document E&M Services using the **SOAP Note** format. SOAP is an acronym that stands for: Subjective, Objective, Assessment, Plan. The **subjective** portion of the note consists of asking the patient questions. It is subjective because the physician must rely on the patient's responses for information. The **objective** portion of the note consists of observing the patient through examination. It is objective because the physician relies on his/her own observations for information. The **assessment** portion of the note consists of the diagnostic process used in order to arrive at a diagnosis. The **plan** portion of the note consists of determining either how to manage the diagnosis, or if additional information is needed to determine a final diagnosis, a plan for further testing and discussing the plan with the patient.

The documentation may be written in a variety of formats, but the SOAP note is the basic format on which most E&M visits are written. The elements of the SOAP note relate directly to CPT E&M components.

! KEY TERMS

SOAP Note—Documentation format taught in medical school.
Subjective—Consists of asking the patient questions.
Objective—Observing the patient through examination.
Assessment—Consists of the process used in order to arrive at a diagnosis.
Plan—Determining how to manage the diagnosis or a plan for further testing to determine a diagnosis.

■ Example of E&M visit documented in the SOAP note format

Subjective: By trade, Mr. Kim, is a 35-year-old welder who was found to have borderline glucose levels during a hospital stay 1 month ago. The levels were higher after meals but never exceeded 200 mg/dL. The patient thinks he might have experienced some frequent urination, but that could be from increased fluid intake. Since his hospital stay, the patient has been concerned about his blood sugar and has started walking 20 minutes at least 5 days/week and reducing his caloric intake. Mr. Kim reports no recent weight changes or changes in appetite. His vision has returned to normal since his corneal transplant. He has not noticed any recent cuts or bruises that are slow to heal. No extremity tingling or numbness. No oral infections. No skin infections. No bladder infections. Normal bowel movements. No shortness of breath, no chest pains. Patient reports his knees hurt from time to time from remote history of athletics, but the pain is controlled with ibuprofen. No depression, slight anxiety concerning healing eye trauma. No other current endocrine symptoms

Example of E&M visit documented in the SOAP note format—cont'd

or disease. Patient is immunosuppressed due to the corneal transplant and reports his medication is preventing rejection. Patient has recent surgical history of corneal transplant without complication. Is immunosuppressed. No other medications. Patient reports paternal grandfather developed type II diabetes over 60. No other diabetic history.

Objective: On exam, head is normocephalic and atraumatic. Neck is supple with no lymphadenopathy. Trachea midline. Pupils are equal, round, and reactive to light and accommodation. Nares are clear. On auscultation, heart has regular rate and rhythm. Patient's abdomen is soft and nontender, positive bowel sounds, no organomegaly, no hernias. External genitalia are normal. All four extremities have full range of motion, positive reflexes. Skin normal.

Assessment and Plan: Mr. Kim had recent elevated blood sugars, but latest test shows high normal. At this time I would not consider him diabetic or prediabetic, given his absence of symptoms and transient blood sugar levels. Mr. Kim should continue his new diet and exercise habits. I gave him a pamphlet today on healthy eating. Mr. Kim should see me every 6 months to monitor his progress and hopefully avoid any disease process. Should his blood sugars start to increase, we will revisit his diagnosis and treatment. At this point, I think Mr. Kim has a moderate risk of developing type II diabetes at some point in the future.

E&M COMPONENTS

Nearly every E&M service has 7 components as its foundation. For many E&M service codes, these components also form the basis for selecting the correct code. For others, it is the absence of these components that are the basis of the code. The 7 components of an E&M service are: history, examination, medical decision making, counseling, coordination of care, nature of presenting problem, and time.

The SOAP note format translates directly into the first three components. **History** describes the subjective portion of a visit. **Examination** is the objective portion of a visit. **Medical Decision Making (MDM)** is the assessment and plan potions of a visit (Fig. 9-1). History, Examination, and MDM are so important to developing an E&M service level that, without them, it is often impossible to describe the service adequately. It would be unusual for documentation of a visit to include history and examination but no medical decision-making. For even basic services, the physician will always ask some question that encompasses history. Because these components are the basic building blocks of any E&M service level, they are referred to as the **key components.**

KEY TERMS

History—Key component that describes the subjective portion of the visit.
Exam—Key component that describes the objective portion of the visit.
Medical Decision Making—Key component that describes the assessment and plan portions of the visit.
Key components—CPT-defined note components that are the basic building blocks of a note: History, Exam, and Medical Decision Making.

| | | Key |
SOAP		component
Subjective	=	History
Objective	=	Examination
Assessment and **P**lan	=	Medical decision making

FIGURE 9-1 The SOAP note format translates directly into the first 3 components: history (the Subjective portion of a visit); examination (the Objective portion of a visit); and medical decision making (the Assessment and Plan portions of a visit).

The next three components are the **contributory components.** Although contributory components do have some bearing on selecting the correct E&M service level, they are not critical and may not exist in every E&M service.

Counseling describes the physician discussing diagnosis and treatment options with the patient. **Coordination of Care** includes ordering diagnostic studies, planning return visits, asking a nurse to complete incidental care, and other associated services. Counseling and Coordination of Care are typically included in the Plan portion of the note.

❗ KEY TERMS

Contributory components—CPT-defined components that often exist but are not necessary to a note: Counseling, Coordination of Care, Nature of Presenting Problem.

Counseling—Contributing component that describes the physician discussing with the patient diagnosis and treatment options.

Coordination of care—Contributing component that includes ordering diagnostic studies, planning return visits, asking a nurse to complete incidental care, and other associated services.

While the other components are often documented in an explicit manner, the **Nature of Presenting Problem** (NOPP) is much more of a conceptual component, describing how many differential diagnoses a presenting problem creates, or the typical outcome for a presenting problem. NOPP is closely related to the concept of **medical necessity.** Most insurance payers will only reimburse specifically covered preventive care services and those services deemed medically necessary. For example, a patient that presents with symptoms of the common cold would not meet the medical necessity requirements for a high level E&M visit because the nature of presenting problem is simple and uncomplicated. However, if the physician also documents the patient's medically induced immunosuppressed state due to regular infusions to treat rheumatoid arthritis, medical necessity for a high level visit may be met since the nature of presenting problem includes the potential of a much more serious illness.

❗ KEY TERMS

Nature of Presenting Problem—Contributing component that is much more of a conceptual component, describing how many differential diagnoses a presenting problem creates, or the typical outcome for a presenting problem.

Medical necessity—Concept closely related to Nature of Presenting Problem, relating to whether the services rendered were necessary to treat the patient's condition effectively.

Time is the seventh component. Time is used for E&M services in a variety of ways (as a contributing factor to component based codes, as the principal component for certain E&M services, and as the primary description of some services. Time as the principal component is described in detail in Chapter 13, Contributing Components & Time. Time as the primary description of some services is addressed later in this chapter.

❗ KEY TERM

Time—Seventh component; the length of the E&M service.

■ CODING METHODS—KEY COMPONENT-BASED CODES

The typical way to think of an E&M service is one that is key component-based, requiring identification of the place or type of service and the key components. As introduced in Chapter 4, and shown here in Figure 9-2, these codes describe the service subcategory and increasing levels of complexity represented

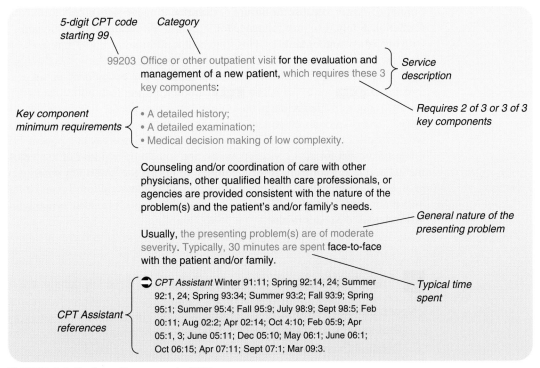

FIGURE 9-2 Code as it appears in CPT.

by increasingly complex *minimum* key components, general nature of the presenting problem, and the typical time spent performing the service.

E&M code descriptions always start with the category or subcategory description. In Figure 9-2, the description of 99201 begins, "Office or other outpatient visit for the evaluation and management of a new patient, which requires these 3 key components." The description identifies this code as part of the Office or Other Outpatient Services category, which requires that the service is rendered in an outpatient setting, most often in a physician's office, and that the patient is new to the practice or has not been seen in the practice for at least three years. Each code in this subcategory (99201-99205) begins with the same description. Review this code series, as well as 99211-99215, in the CPT manual.

The key components are listed next, always in this order – history, examination, and medical decision making. Notice that each component includes a type of the component, such as a problem focused history, or comprehensive exam. As shown in the CPT manual, 99201 requires a *problem focused* history, a *problem focused* examination, and *straightforward* medical decision making. As shown in Figure 9-2, code 99203 requires a *detailed* history, a *detailed* examination, and medical decision making of *low complexity*. These component types are the minimum level of the component required to report the E&M code. A service that can be described as having *expanded problem focused* history, a *detailed* examination, and medical decision making of *low complexity* does not meet the minimum requirements to report 99203, because the history is not detailed. That service does meet the minimum requirements for 99202, because it includes *at least* an *expanded problem focused* history, an *expanded problem focused* examination, and *straightforward* medical decision making. It is acceptable that the examination and medical decision making *exceed* the requirements for the code. These types are addressed in detail in later chapters.

The next element of the code description is usually, "Counseling and/or coordination of care with other providers or agencies are provided consistent with the nature of the problem(s) and the patient's and/or family's needs." This statement is general because the counseling and coordination of care included in 99201 as provided by a dermatologist will differ significantly from the same services provided by a urologist. Because counseling and coordination of care are contributing components, there is no minimum requirement for them in the code description.

The last paragraph of the code description includes a reference to the presenting problem and typical time. The presenting problem reference for 99201 is, "Usually, the presenting problem(s) are self limited or minor." Again, because the nature of the presenting problem is only a contributing factor, this is informational only. The time reference for 99201 is, "Physicians typically spend 10 minutes face-to-face with the patient and/or family." This statement is informational and may guide the coder toward a correct code, but it is not required.

In Chapters 5 to 8, the E&M categories that are key component–based are marked with either a 2 of 3 icon `2 of 3` or a 3 of 3 icon `3 of 3`. In the CPT manual, notice the first part of the description for 99201 ends, "which requires these three key components." Compare this with the description for 99213, "Office or other outpatient visit for the evaluation and management of an established patient, which requires *at least 2 of these 3* key components." Some key component–based codes require the minimum be met for all 3 key components, and some only require 2 of the 3 component minimums be met. If only 2 key components are required, disregard the lowest key component. Every key component–based code includes this information in the code description. It can be helpful to highlight this information in each code description with two different colors, such as highlighting all 3 of 3 codes in yellow and 2 of 3 codes in blue.

Example of how to select correct code when all three key component minimums required

New patient office visit
  Problem focused History
  Detailed Examination
  Medical Decision Making of moderate complexity
Starting with 99201, consider whether all of the key component requirements are met for each level.

	History	Examination	Medical Decision Making	Meet Requirements?
99201	**Problem focused**	Problem focused	Straightforward	**Yes**
99202	Expanded problem focused	Expanded problem focused	Straightforward	No
99203	Detailed	**Detailed**	Low	No
99204	Comprehensive	Comprehensive	**Moderate**	No
99205	Comprehensive	Comprehensive	High	No

The highest level where all three components are met is 99201. Even though the medical decision making qualifies for 99204, and the examination qualifies for 99203, the history only meets the *minimum* requirements for 99201. So, the highest level where *all three* elements meet the *minimum* requirements is 99201. It is acceptable that the examination and medical decision making are far higher than the minimum requirements for 99201. All three must be met.

The following example illustrates how to select the correct code when the category requires only 2 of the 3 key component minimums. Notice as well that the key component types in this example are the same as in the previous example but result in a very different level selection. Levels of different E&M categories do not necessarily require the same key component minimums. Always consider the key components for the specific category selected.

Example of how to select correct code when category requires only two of three key component minimums

Established patient office visit

    Problem focused History

    Detailed Examination

    Medical Decision Making of moderate complexity

Starting with 99212 (99211 does not require physician presence), consider whether all of the key component requirements are met for each level. Problem focused history is the lowest element, so disregard it. Only the examination and medical decision making are considered for this visit.

	History	Examination Making	Medical Decision	Meet Requirements?
99212	**Problem focused**	Problem focused	Straightforward	Yes
99213	Expanded problem focused	Expanded problem focused	Low	Yes
99214	Detailed	**Detailed**	**Moderate**	Yes
99215	Comprehensive	Comprehensive	High	No

The highest level where at least two components are met is 99214. Report 99214 for this service.

CRITICAL THINKING

Why do some E&M types require only the minimums for 2 of 3 key components to be met?

■ CODING METHODS—CODE SPECIFIC SERVICE

Key component–based codes are usually associated with the term E&M, but there are many codes in the CPT Evaluation and Management chapter that are not key component–based. These codes utilize directions specific to the category or code to select the correct code. These codes are in categories described in Chapters 5 to 8 that are *not* marked as 2 of 3 `2 of 3` or 3 of 3 `3 of 3`. Instructions to select these codes are included in those chapters.

These codes are defined by the service provided—either the service was provided, or it was not—without regard to the key components. Code 99288, *Physician direction of emergency medical systems (EMS) emergency care, advanced life support,* is a good example. If this code describes a service, then the physician-directed EMS care includes directing advanced life support. It does not matter whether the physician collected any history about the patient (although he/she probably did). It does not matter that the physician could not complete an examination because the patient was not present. It does not matter how long the physician directed care. The only requirement for this code is that the work described was performed. Newborn care, 99460-99463, is another example of codes that do not require key component minimums or any specific time. Review the requirements to report these codes in the CPT manual.

Some codes defined by the service provided include a required time component. For example, code 99360, *Physician standby service, requiring prolonged physician attendance, each 30 minutes (e.g., operative standby, standby for frozen section, for cesarean/high risk delivery, for monitoring EEG).* Not only must standby services occur, but the service must also last at least 30 minutes to report the code.

Time can also be the element that differentiates codes in a series. The two codes in the Discharges Services category, 99238 and 92239, differ by the time spent performing the service: 30 minutes or less for 99238, and more than 30 minutes for 99239. Telephone services are also defined by the amount of time spent: 99441—5 to 10 minutes, 99442—11 to 20 minutes, and 99443—21 to 30 minutes. The time in these codes increases, but only one code is reported.

Some time-based codes build on the previous code in the series and are reported in addition to the first code. For Critical Care Services (99291–99292), 99291—first 30 to 74 minutes are always reported. If additional time is spent, 99292—each additional 30 minutes, may be reported *in addition* to 99291. Code 99292 is designated in CPT as an add-on code (+), which means it is always reported with a parent code. Prolonged Physician Service with Direct Patient Contact (99354–99357) is also only reported with a parent code from the listed E&M categories. Notice as well that 99354 or 99356 is reported as the first add-on code, by place of service, and then 99355 or 99357 is added.

●●● SUMMARY

- E&M services have 7 components.
- The 3 key components are: history, examination, and medical decision making.
- The 3 contributing components are: counseling, coordination of care, and nature of presenting problem.
- Time is the 7th component.
- Key component–based code descriptions include the place or type of service, key component minimums, typical nature of presenting problem, and typical time spent.
- Key component–based codes require either 2 of 3 or 3 of 3 key component minimums to be met.
- Some codes are not key component–based and include code-specific instructions. These codes may require only a specific service or may have a time requirement as well.

Chapter Review Exercises

1. Name the 7 components and identify them as:
   a. Key components
   b. Contributory components
   c. Seventh component

2. Identify 3 E&M categories not described in the chapter that are not key component–based.

Questions 3–10: For the following services:
   A. Identify whether the code requires 2 of 3 key component minimums, 3 of 3 key component minimums, or is a code-specific service.
   B. Select the correct specific code. You may need to refer to Chapters 5 to 8 to select the correct E&M category.

3. New patient office visit documented with detailed history, detailed exam, and medical decision making of high complexity.

4. Established patient office visit documented with detailed history, detailed exam, and medical decision making of high complexity.

5. Hospital admission documented with comprehensive history, comprehensive exam, and medical decision making of high complexity.

6. Hospital rounding visit on the third day of the patient's stay documented with detailed examination, medical decision making of high complexity. No history was documented.

7. An outpatient consultation documented with detailed history, problem focused examination, and medical decision making of high complexity.

8. A family practice physician sees an established patient in the local emergency room and documents an expanded problem focused history, an expanded problem focused examination, and medical decision making of low complexity.

9. A patient is discharged from a nursing facility. The physician documents spending 45 minutes with the patient.

10. A physician spends 25 minutes supervising a hospice patient's complex multidisciplinary care.

CASE STUDY

Revisit the Case Study from Chapter 3. Assign the correct E&M code for each encounter. Assume that all services are documented. (Do not assign any modifiers, just the E&M code for the visit.)

Henry Kim is a 35-year-old welder in Grand Island, Nebraska. While at work welding, a metal splinter became lodged in Henry's eye. Henry went to the emergency room. Henry complained of pain from the splinter as well as a feeling of lightheadedness and shortness of breath. Dr. Hansen saw Mr. Kim and documented a detailed history. Dr. Hansen also completed a detailed examination of Henry and determined that his non-pain symptoms were due to hyperventilation secondary to the accident at work. The physician then examined Henry's eye with a slit lamp and saw the splinter lodged in the cornea. Dr. Hansen carefully removed the splinter from Henry's eye, bandaged it, and sent him home with aftercare instructions. The physician completed medical decision making of moderate complexity.

1. Dr. Hansen's visit

As the next few weeks went by, Henry's vision became increasingly blurry, his eye watered continuously, and he continued to experience pain. Henry went to a local ophthalmologist, Dr. Wheaton, for further treatment and was new to the practice. Dr. Wheaton determined that the emergency physician did not remove the entire metal splinter from Henry's cornea. He completed a comprehensive history and expanded problem focused exam. It was the ophthalmologist's opinion the cornea had been permanently scarred and the only treatment that would restore Henry's vision would be a corneal transplant. His medical decision making was of moderate level complexity.

2. Dr. Wheaton's visit

Because corneal transplants are an expensive treatment, Henry's workers' compensation insurance carrier wanted him to have a second opinion from another ophthalmologist, who also happened to perform corneal transplants, at the academic medical center in Omaha, Nebraska, Dr. Samson. Henry traveled to Omaha, about 3 hours away, to see the second ophthalmologist, who agreed that a transplant was necessary. Henry was also new to Dr. Samson's practice. Because he had complete documentation from Dr. Wheaton, Dr. Samson completed an expanded problem focused history and an expanded problem focused exam. His medical decision making was of high complexity.

3. Dr. Samson's visit

Surprisingly, a cornea donation was available that was a match for Henry, and surgery was scheduled for early the next morning.

Henry had surgery the next day, and the transplant was a success. During his preoperative work-up, Henry was found to have borderline glucose levels. Dr. Samson asked an endocrinologist, Dr. Lester, to evaluate Henry for diabetes while he was an inpatient. Dr. Lester saw Henry and completed a comprehensive history, comprehensive exam, and had medical decision making of moderate complexity. Dr. Lester completed his note in the shared medical record. He determined that Henry did not have diabetes but should be monitored regularly when he returned home and made some recommendations about diet and exercise. Henry was discharged home after 2 days.

4. Dr. Lester's visit

CASE STUDY—cont'd

Henry saw his ophthalmologist in Grand Island at regular intervals to find out how well the graft was healing. Everything looked fine, although the typical postoperative care for a corneal transplant lasts at least a year. During the postoperative period, Henry saw an endocrinologist in Grand Island, Dr. Bellkey, for a recheck of his glucose levels. Dr. Bellkey documented a comprehensive history, a detailed exam, and came to medical decision making of moderate complexity. She thought Henry was doing well and asked him to return in a year for a follow-up visit.

5. Dr. Bellkey's visit

Henry returned to see Dr. Bellkey in a year. She once again completed a comprehensive history, a detailed exam, and came to medical decision making of moderate complexity. She once again thought Henry was doing well but noticed he had not seen his internist for a general check-up for many years and recommended he go in for a physical.

6. Dr. Bellkey's second visit

Henry took her advice and scheduled a physical with his family practice physician, Dr. Johnson. Dr. Johnson noted it had been 5 years since she last saw Henry. Dr. Johnson completed a comprehensive preventive medicine evaluation that included an age- and gender-appropriate history, examination, counseling, risk factor reduction interventions, and she ordered a general lab panel to check his cholesterol, glucose, and overall health. Henry appeared to be in good health, and Dr. Johnson was pleased that his eyes had healed well and his vision was back to normal.

7. Dr. Johnson's visit

History

Chapter Outline

LEARNING OUTCOMES

On completion of this chapter, you will be able to:

1. Enumerate the types of History.
2. Differentiate the four elements of History.
3. Identify in an Evaluation and Management (E&M) note the History of Present Illness.
4. Identify in an E&M note the Review of Systems.
5. Identify in an E&M note the Past, Family, and Social History.
6. Compare Review of Systems and Past History.
7. Identify the correct History type.

KEY TERMS

Associated Signs and
  Symptoms
Chief Complaint
Context
Element
Family History
History

History of Present Illness
  (HPI)
Location
Modifying Factors
History
Past, Family, Social
  History (PSFH)

Quality
Review of Systems (ROS)
Severity
SOAP note
Social History
Timing

History is the first of the 3 key components required to report component-based E&M codes. This key component describes the physician's work collecting subjective information from the patient. That information includes the Chief Complaint, History of Present Illness, Review of Systems, and Past, Family, Social History. The level of documentation of these elements determines which of the four History types is correct. This chapter describes History as defined by CPT, which differs from the often-used Medicare Documentation Guidelines. Additional information on History as defined by those Guidelines is included in Chapter 15.

Focus Questions

What element is required for every type of History?

What do coders mean when they say "fish"?

How does History relate to a SOAP note?

If the patient answers a question negatively, does it count?

HISTORY COMPONENT OVERVIEW

The History component of an E&M visit correlates to the Subjective portion of the SOAP note. This is information the physician collects from the patient verbally and is a reflection of the patient's memory and perceptions. The physician collects subjective information to support a diagnostic assessment. That subjective information develops into the four **elements** of the History component—Chief Complaint, History of Present Illness, Review of Systems, and Past, Family, Social History (Fig. 10-1).

! KEY TERM

Elements—Building blocks of a Key Component.

Although the physician uses the patient's answers to develop a diagnosis and treatment plan, it is the evidence that the physician asked a question, not the patient's answer, that is important to selecting the correct E&M code. E&M codes report the physician's effort, not the patient's diagnosis, much like all CPT codes represent the work performed, not the condition treated. Because the coder is looking for evidence of physician effort, not the patient's diagnosis, both positive and negative answers count toward the code.

■ Examples of negative answers to History questions

These answers are evidence that the physician asked a question about the patient's condition, and credit is given to the element.

History of Present Illness
- The patient cannot remember when the pain began.
- The patient has not taken any antacids to try and control his heartburn symptoms.
- The patient does not report any numbness or tingling when the pain occurs.

Review of Systems
- The patient has no neurological symptoms.
- The patient has been sleeping well and has not lost any weight suddenly.
- Cardiovascular system is negative.

Past, Family, Social History
- No surgical history.
- There is no history of stroke in the patient's family.
- The patient does not smoke.

CHIEF COMPLAINT

The **Chief Complaint** is the foundation of every E&M note. It is a simple concept and probably the most important to E&M coding. The Chief Complaint is the patient's presenting problem in his/her

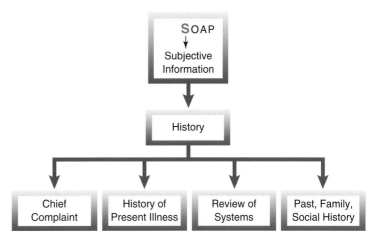

FIGURE 10-1 Subjective information develops into the four elements of the History component: Chief Complaint; History of Present Illness; Review of Systems; and Past, Family, and Social History.

own words, and the remainder of the E&M note references the Chief Complaint. If the note does not include a Chief Complaint, then it is not possible to determine the correct E&M code. All components and their elements are considered as they affect the Chief Complaint. For example, there cannot be a problem pertinent History of Present Illness if there is no problem listed.

! KEY TERM

Chief Complaint—Patient's presenting problem; the foundation of every E&M note.

■ Examples of a Chief Complaint

- The patient presents today with shoulder pain.
- Chief Complaint: Sore throat
- "I feel dizzy when I stand up."
- Med check

 CRITICAL THINKING

Why is "follow-up" a valid Chief Complaint?

■ HISTORY OF PRESENT ILLNESS

The physician asks the patient questions about the Chief Complaint, which then develops into a **History of Present Illness (HPI).** The HPI is the story of the patient's Chief Complaint from the first signs of the condition to the current visit or from the last time the patient saw the physician for the condition to the current visit. CPT includes two types of HPI, brief and extended (Fig. 10-2). These HPI types do not have any additional definition in CPT, but the questions the physician may ask the patient describe seven elements of HPI—location, quality, severity, timing, context, modifying factors, and associated signs and symptoms. Table 10.1 describes these areas. The Medicare documentation guidelines include an eighth element, duration, which is addressed in Chapter 15.

! KEY TERM

History of Present Illness (HPI)—The story of the patient's Chief Complaint from the first signs of the condition to the current visit or from the last time the patient saw the physician for the condition to the current visit.

Example of an HPI

Although typical HPI statements do not usually include all of the elements, this is an example of an HPI: "The patient is an otherwise healthy 10-year-old boy, well known to the practice, who presents with a history of increasingly sore throat and difficulty swallowing. He describes the soreness as scratchy and feels it is worse in the morning. He has tried gargling warm salt water, with little effect. His mother reports he has also had a low-grade fever for 2 days. There have been children in his class out sick with strep throat in recent weeks."

- Chief Complaint: sore throat
- Elements:
  - Location—throat
  - Quality – scratchy
  - Severity—increasingly
  - Timing—worse in the morning
  - Context—schoolmates recently sick with strep throat
  - Modifying factors— gargling warm salt water
  - Associated signs and symptoms—difficulty swallowing, low-grade fever

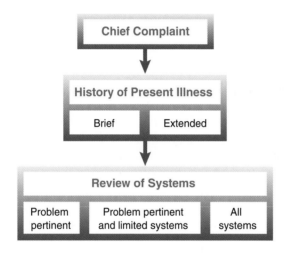

FIGURE 10-2 The Chief Complaint develops into an HPI. CPT includes two HPI: Brief and Extended.

TABLE 10.1 History of Present Illness Elements

Element	Definition	Examples
Location	Anatomical body part	Right leg Throat LUQ All over Abdomen
Quality	How the patient characterizes the Chief Complaint (usually an adjective for the Chief Complaint)	Sharp, dull, throbbing, or radiating (pain) Persistent Dry/wet (cough)
Severity	How bad, or how difficult it is to endure the Chief Complaint	Pain on a scale Worse than... Mild, moderate, severe Better/worse So bad that is causes some effect

TABLE 10.1   History of Present Illness Elements—cont'd

Element	Definition	Examples
Timing	Frequency of the Chief Complaint, or patterns when the Chief Complaint occurs	Every morning All the time Intermittent Usually in the evening
Context	Conditions that cause the Chief Complaint to occur Conditions present in the patient's environment when it occurs	When the patient stands up The patient fell When the patient pets her dog If the patient runs more than 20 minutes Only when the patient is sleeping
Modifying factors	What the patient has done to try and resolve the problem	Ice and ibuprofen Takes as many as 6 antacid tablets 3 ×day Stretches when standing Better after 30 minutes rest Has not tried anything
Associated signs and symptoms Numbness	Other conditions that occur with the Chief Complaint	Nausea and vomiting Pain Blurred vision No other complaints

■ REVIEW OF SYSTEMS

After identifying the Chief Complaint and developing an HPI, the physician asks questions to determine whether the patient has any other issues that might affect the Chief Complaint. Because the physician records these questions by organ system, this section of the note is the **Review of Systems (ROS).** CPT includes three types of ROS—problem pertinent system review, problem pertinent system and limited additional system review, and all systems (see Fig. 10-2). There is no CPT definition of "problem pertinent and limited additional system review." However, because the next level requires a review of all systems, the coder may presume that this level includes 2 to 13 systems reviewed. CPT recognizes 14 systems for ROS, which are listed in Table 10.2.

❗ KEY TERM

Review of Systems (ROS)—The physician asks questions to determine whether the patient has any other issues that might affect the Chief Complaint. Recorded by organ system.

■ Example of a ROS

For the young patient with a sore throat, a typical ROS would be, "The patient has been sleeping well and has not had any recent weight loss. No report of itching eyes. His nose has started to run today. CV negative. His mother says his breathing has not been labored. No achiness. No rashes. The patient has mild environmental allergies and has not recently been exposed to any new allergens."

• Constitutional—sleeping well; no recent weight loss
• Eyes—no report of itching eyes
• ENMT—runny nose
• Cardiovascular— negative
• Respiratory—breathing is not labored

Continued

Example of a ROS—cont'd

- Musculoskeletal—no achiness
- Integumentary—no rashes
- Allergic/immunological—mild environmental allergies

TABLE 10.2   CPT Recognized Organ Systems for Review of Systems

System	Example
Constitutional	Sleep Fever Weight/eating patterns
Eyes	Watery Itchy No changes Recent change in prescription
Ears, Nose, Mouth, Throat (ENMT)	Ringing in ears Runny nose Postnasal drip Patient reports a dry mouth No tooth pain Sore throat Itchy throat
Cardiovascular	Heart palpitations No chest pain Occasional flushing
Respiratory	Shortness of breath after climbing a flight of stairs Persistent cough
Gastrointestinal (GI)	Regular bowel movements Heartburn No stomach pains
Genitourinary (GU)	No blood observed in urine Patient reports a slow urine stream Vaginal discharge not associated with menstrual cycle
Musculoskeletal	Aches Specific pain Stiff joints
Integumentary (skin and/or breast)	Rashes Hives Slow healing wound Nipple discharge
Neurological	Fainting Seizures Headache
Psychiatric	Depression Anxiety Is not currently being treated for psychiatric condition
Endocrine	Diabetes control Polyuria Excessive sweating
Hematological/Lymphatic	Bruising Bleeding Chronic swollen lymph nodes
Allergic/immunological	Allergies control, current allergen problems HIV status with control

Questions asked in the ROS refer to the current status of a system or condition, not whether the patient has had a condition previously, which is recorded as past history. The words "history of" always denote past history, not ROS, regardless of the section of the note in which the physician records the comment. For example, compare "The patient has a history of diabetes" (Past History) with "The patient's diabetes is well-controlled," (ROS—Endocrine).

■ PAST, FAMILY, SOCIAL HISTORY

Past, Family, Social History is abbreviated **PFSH** and pronounced "fish" by many coders. PFSH describes the patient's history and environmental factors that might cause or affect the Chief Complaint or influence the patient's recovery. Past history includes a wide range of information that encompasses what is usually considered patient history. Family history is not a description of the family members but, instead, is a review of the family's past history and current conditions as they relate to the patient's Chief Complaint. Social history should always be age-appropriate. The social history for a child will be markedly different from social history for an adult. For example, a physician will assume an infant does not smoke, but it would be pertinent to note whether the infant is exposed to second-hand smoke.

! KEY TERM

Past, Family, Social History (PFSH)—Describes the patient's history and environmental factors that might cause or affect the Chief Complaint or influence the patient's recovery.

Table 10.3 lists the major elements of PFSH. Only one item must be documented to count the PFSH element. At least one item from each PFSH element must be documented to count all three histories. CPT includes two types of PFSH—pertinent or complete. The coder may presume pertinent is one or two of the history elements, and complete is all three.

■ Example of a PFSH

For the patient with a sore throat, this might be a typical PFSH, "The patient has a history upper respiratory infections but does not report any regular history of throat infections. No prior hospitalizations or surgeries. The patient has environmental allergies; no known drug allergies. Immunizations are current. The patient lives with his parents and two siblings, none of whom have been ill with similar symptoms in the recent past. The patient is active in soccer and attends 5th grade regularly."

- Past history—upper respiratory infections (medical); no throat infections (medical); no prior hospitalizations or surgeries (surgical); environmental allergies, NKDA (allergies); immunizations current.
- Family history—No one in the family has been ill with similar symptoms.
- Social history—Lives with his parents and two siblings; active in soccer; 5th grade.

✳ Communicating With Medical Providers

Many physicians document past medical history, past surgical history, previous hospitalizations, immunizations, and other past history information. They then expect each of these sections to "be a point" under PFSH. Unfortunately, all this history is considered Past History. This is a good time to discuss with the physician how documentation for billing should not cause unnecessary documentation that is not medically necessary. The physician should document only those elements of Past History that have bearing on the Chief Complaint or the patient's recovery.

TABLE 10.3 Past, Family, Social History Elements

Past History	Family History	Social History
Medical history	Medical events in the family	Past and current activities
Surgical history	Family health status	Marital status

Prior hospitalization	Cause of death of immediate family members	Living arrangements
		    At home with his mother
		    With a roommate
		    In a shelter

Medication list	Diseases related to the Chief Complaint	Employment status
Allergies	Hereditary diseases	Drug, alcohol, tobacco use/ frequency
Immunizations Dietary status		Education Sexual history

■ FOUR TYPES OF HISTORY

There are four types of History—Problem Focused, Expanded Problem Focused, Detailed, and Comprehensive. The History type depends on the various levels of the four History elements. Table 10.4 describes the four types of History and their related element minimums.

Notice that occasionally two types of History require the same element level. When this occurs, the higher History type is credited. For example, both Detailed and Comprehensive require an extended HPI, so the Comprehensive type is credited.

Review the History presented throughout the chapter for the sample patient. There is a Chief Complaint present—Sore throat. For HPI, CPT does not define a brief versus extended HPI, but with five of the eight possible HPI elements identified, we can probably describe this HPI as extended. With more systems reviewed than the problem pertinent system, but fewer than all of the systems reviews, the ROS is problem pertinent with limited additional systems. The physician provided some type of information for all three types of history, so the PFSH is complete. Table 10.5 summarizes the History elements for the sample patient.

TABLE 10.4 History Types and Element Minimums for Each Type

History Type	Chief Complaint	HPI	ROS	PFSH
Problem Focused	Required	Brief	None	None
Expanded Problem Focused	Required	Brief	Problem pertinent	None
Detailed	Required	Extended	Problem pertinent and limited additional systems	Problem pertinent
Comprehensive	Required	Extended	All systems	Complete

TABLE 10.5   Summary History for Sample Patient

History Type	Chief Complaint	HPI	ROS	PFSH
Problem Focused	Required	Brief	None	None
Expanded Problem Focused	Required	Brief	Problem pertinent	None
Detailed	**Required**	**Extended**	**Problem pertinent and limited additional systems**	Problem pertinent
Comprehensive	Required	Extended	All systems	**Complete**

Similar to the minimum requirements for selecting a key component–based E&M code, the minimum element levels must be met in order to select a History type. Select the History based on the lowest-level element documented. While the Chief Complaint, HPI, and PFSH were all documented to the Comprehensive History level, the ROS was documented only to the Detailed History level, so the overall History type for this visit is Detailed.

SUMMARY

- The History component comprises the Subjective portion of a SOAP format note.
- History elements are proof that the physician asked a question, not whether the patient's answer was positive.
- The four elements of History are Chief Complaint, History of Present Illness (HPI), Review of Systems (ROS), and Past, Family, Social History (PFSH).
- Every E&M visit must have a Chief Complaint.
- There are seven elements of HPI specified in CPT—location, quality, severity, timing, context, modifying factors, and associated signs and symptoms.
- There are 14 systems considered for ROS.
- ROS represents the current status of systems and related conditions.
- PFSH includes past, family, and social histories.
- Past history includes many elements, including medical and surgical history, medication list, immunizations, and allergies.
- The four History types are Problem Focused, Expanded Problem Focused, Detailed, and Comprehensive.
- All listed minimum element requirements must be met to select a History type. The lowest documented element will determine the History type.

Chapter Review Exercises

1. Match one of the seven HPI elements to each of the following documentation excerpts (location, quality, severity, timing, context, modifying factors, associated signs and symptoms):

   A. Knee pain

   B. Constant pain

   C. Pain is rated 7 on a 10-point scale

   D. The pain is worse in the evening

   E. The pain is worse when standing for more than a few minutes or when using stairs

   F. The patient has tried acetaminophen, ibuprofen, and Alleve, with no significant relief

   G. When the pain is the worst, the patient's knee is also warm to the touch and slightly reddened

2. Match one of the seven HPI elements to each of the following documentation excerpts (location, quality, severity, timing, context, modifying factors, associated signs & symptoms):

   A. Cough (lungs)

   B. The cough is worse than usual

   C. The patient does not notice anything that triggers the cough

   D. The cough is productive

   E. The cough is not accompanied by any upper respiratory symptoms

   F. The cough is relieved temporarily by OTC cough medicine

   G. The cough is intermittent, seeming to be better some days, worse others

3. Identify the seven systems reviewed in the following documentation excerpt
   Chief Complaint: Right knee pain
   Review of Systems: Constitutional: negative. The patient reports no tingling or numbness in either leg. No pain in the left knee. Cardiovascular/Respiratory: negative. No changes to the skin around the knee. No unusual bleeding recently.

4. Identify the eight systems reviewed in the following documentation excerpt:
   Chief Complaint: cough
   Review of Systems: Patient reports no recent fever, no weight changes, no trouble sleeping. Eyes: negative. ENT: negative. Cardiovascular: no reported chest pain. Respiratory: positive cough with production. No shortness of breath. No rashes or hives. Patient has a history of sinus headaches, but none recently. No reported allergies.

5. Identify whether the following statements are ROS or Past History:

   A. Patient has a history of diabetes type II

   B. Patient reports diabetes type II, well controlled by daily glucophage

   C. Patient reports intermittent chest pain on exertion

   D. History of MI

   E. Asthma

   F. Childhood asthma

   G. Exercise-induced asthma, resolves easily with rescue inhaler

   H. Wears glasses

6. Identify whether the following documentation excerpt includes past, family, and/or social history:

   Chief Complaint: right knee pain

   No joint surgery. NKDA. Sister had knee replacement 4 years ago. Patient is a retired factory assembly worker. Lives at home with his spouse. No history of tobacco use. Drinks one or two beers in the evening.

7. Identify whether the following documentation excerpt includes past, family, and/or social history:

   Chief Complaint: cough

   Immunizations current. Tonsils removed two years ago. Patient's sister has had bronchitis.

8. Identify whether the following documentation excerpt includes past, family, and/or social history.

   Chief Complaint: Depression

   History of DVT. Hypercholesterolemia. Appendectomy in remote past. NKDA. The patient has two sisters.

9. Assign the History type for documentation that includes:
   Chief Complaint
   Brief HPI
   Problem Pertinent ROS
   No PFSH

10. Assign the History type for documentation that includes:
    Chief Complaint
    Extended HPI
    All systems ROS
    No PFSH

CASE STUDY

Revisit the Case Study presented in Chapter 3. Read the following documentation sample and answer the questions below:

Patient presents with report of foreign object in right eye. Henry Kim is a 35-year-old welder. While at work welding, a metal splinter became lodged in his eye. Henry presents to the ED today complaining of pain from the splinter as well as a feeling of light-headedness and shortness of breath. The incident occurred at approximately 1400 hours this afternoon. The pain is an 8 out of 10. Patient reports no constitutional symptoms. Vision is blurred. The patient's mouth feels dry. Feels like his heart is racing. Previously reported shortness of breath. Patient is not nauseated. No other pain in the head and neck. Patient did not notice any debris that hit or became lodged in his face or arms. No headache. No surgical history. Previous history of splinter in eye. NKDA. No daily medications. Patient lives alone.

1. Identify the Chief Complaint.
2. Identify the elements of HPI.
3. Identify the HPI type. (For this exercise, consider 1–3 elements = Brief, 4–7 elements = Extended.)
4. Identify the systems of review.
5. Identify the problem pertinent system.
6. Identify the ROS type.
7. Identify the elements of PFSH.
8. Identify the PFSH type.
9. Identify the History type.

11

Exam

Chapter Outline

I. Exam Component Overview

II. Body Areas and Organ Systems

III. Examination Formatting

IV. Exam Types

LEARNING OUTCOMES

On completion of this chapter, you will be able to:

1. Count the CPT-defined body areas.
2. Count the CPT-defined organ systems.
3. Identify the types of Exam.
4. Recognize the different ways Exam is documented.

KEY TERMS

Auscultation	Inspection	Percussion
Body area	Palpation	Organ system
Exam		

Exam is the second of the three key components required to report component-based Evaluation and Management (E&M) codes. This key component describes the physician's work of collecting objective information by examining the patient. Exam elements are identified as either body areas or organ systems. The level of Exam documentation determines which of the four Exam types is correct. This chapter describes Exam as defined by CPT, which differs from the popular Medicare Documentation Guidelines. Additional information on Exam as defined by those Guidelines is included in Chapter 15.

Focus Questions

What portion of the SOAP note represents the Exam key component?

What observational methods will the physician use to collect Exam data?

How is a thyroid exam counted?

■ EXAM COMPONENT OVERVIEW

Following the SOAP note format, the Exam component of an E&M visit correlates to the objective portion of the note (Fig. 11-1). This is information the physician collects through personal observation using **inspection**, **auscultation**, **palpation**, **percussion**, and symptom-specific testing. Inspection includes a variety of ways in which the physician visualizes or observes the patient's anatomy and body habitus. Auscultation is the act of listening to a part of the body. Palpation is touching the body. Percussion results from tapping a body part and listening to the result. The physician may also obtain objective information through other specific testing, such as eliciting reflexes or administering a psychiatric evaluation.

❗ KEY TERMS

Inspection—A variety of ways in which the physician visualizes or observes the patient's anatomy and body habitus.
Auscultation—The act of listening to a part of the body.
Palpation—Touching the body.
Percussion—Tapping a body part and listening to the result.

 CRITICAL THINKING

If a physician asks a patient specific questions to complete a psychiatric exam, why is this information considered an objective exam and not part of the subjective History?

■ BODY AREAS AND ORGAN SYSTEMS

CPT recognizes a set of body areas and a set of organ systems for describing the physical exam. Table 11.1 lists the defined body areas and organ systems. Credit each organ system or body area only once, regardless of the number of ways the physician examines an organ system or body area.

Typically, do not mix body areas and organ systems when counting exam elements to avoid double counting an organ system. For example, if cardiovascular (organ system) is counted because the physician palpated the carotid pulse, legs (body area—extremity) are not counted if the physician also observes peripheral edema. The exception to crossing between body areas and organ systems is a thyroid examination. Notice that there is not a defined endocrine organ system. The only way to capture a thyroid exam is to count it as neck. The example below refers to an examination for the sample patient from Chapter 10 who presented with a sore throat.

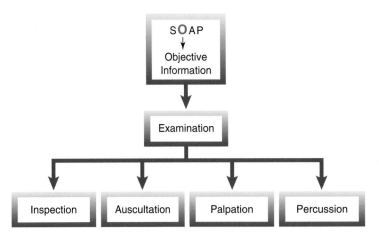

FIGURE 11-1 The Exam component of an E&M visit correlates to the objective portion of the note; it is information the physician collects through personal observation using inspection, auscultation, palpation, percussion, and symptom-specific testing.

TABLE 11.1   CPT-Defined Body Areas and Organ Systems Used to Describe the Physical Exam

CPT-Defined Body Areas	CPT-Defined Organ Systems
Head, including the face	Eyes
Neck	Ears, nose, mouth, and throat
Chest, including breasts and axilla	Cardiovascular
Abdomen	Respiratory
Genitalia, groin, buttocks	Gastrointestinal
Back	Genitourinary
Each extremity	Musculoskeletal
	Skin
	Neurological
	Psychiatric
	Hematological/lymphatic/immunological

■ Example of an organ system–based examination

This is an organ system—based examination for the patient from Chapter 10 who presented with a sore throat.

Patient is a 10-year-old boy.

Chief Complaint: Sore throat

Examination:

Patient is afebrile. No respiratory distress. Pharyngeal exam reveals general erythema, no exudates, minor swelling. Uvula is midline. Upon palpation, cervical lymph nodes are enlarged and tender. Gastrointestinal examination reveals no splenomegaly.

The most common situation in which to identify the exam by body area is for trauma. A patient received in an Emergency Department following trauma is usually examined by body area, head to toe.

■ Example of a body area–based examination

Patient is a 28-year-old male restrained driver in a motor vehicle collision. Patient's car was T-boned on the passenger side by another car.

Head: Atraumatic, normocephalic. Dentition intact. GCS 14.

Neck: Trachea deviated right of midline. No edema. No hematoma. Cervical spine intact.

Chest: Decreased breath sounds on the left side. Reduced chest wall expansion unilaterally. Suspected rib fracture and subcutaneous air.

Abdomen: Diffusely tender on palpation. Positive bowel sounds.

Genitalia, groin, buttocks: Normal rectal tone. No gross deformity.

Back: Atraumatic.

Extremities: Moves all extremities spontaneously and on request. Multiple lacerations present on bilateral arms. No pulsatile bleeding.

■ EXAMINATION FORMATTING

There are two basic formats for the exam note—paragraph and titles. In the paragraph format, the physician records the examination as a narrative, as in the SOAP note format. In titles, the physician documents a title, such as Neck or Cardiovascular, and then follows it with a brief comment. Exam elements can be more difficult to discern in the paragraph format. The titles format may seem more straightforward, but be careful not to be misled by the titles.

Example of a narrative format examination

Patient is a 10-year-old boy.
  Chief Complaint: Sore throat
  Examination:
  Patient is afebrile. Eyes clear. RRR. No respiratory distress. Pharyngeal exam reveals general erythema, no exudates, minor swelling. Uvula is midline. Upon palpation, cervical lymph nodes are enlarged and tender. Abdominal exam reveals no splenomegaly.

Example of a titles format examination

Patient is a 10-year-old boy.
Chief Complaint: Sore throat
Examination:
General: Patient is afebrile.
Head: Atraumatic, normocephalic. Eyes clear.
ENMT: Generalized erythema, no exudates, minor swelling. Uvula is midline.
Neck: Lymph nodes are enlarged and tender. Trachea midline.
CV: RRR.
Respiratory: Normal.
Abdomen: No splenomegaly.

 CRITICAL THINKING

How should "afebrile" be counted as a body area? As an organ system?

If the physician uses the title format, assign the information in the comment to the correct organ system or body area, regardless of the title. For example, "Neurologic: Normal sensation. Cranial nerves II–XII within normal limits. Normal affect." Examination of sensation and cranial nerves is appropriately assigned to the neurological system. However, "affect" is part of a psychiatric exam. So, although there is only one title, the physician examined two organ systems, and both should be counted.

■ EXAM TYPES

There are four types of Exam—Problem Focused, Expanded Problem Focused, Detailed, and Comprehensive (Fig 11-2). Table 11.2 describes the four types of Exam and the corresponding CPT definitions.
Unfortunately, CPT does not provide clear direction on how to determine whether the documented exam meets these definitions. CPT does not articulate what constitutes a limited or extended exam. A

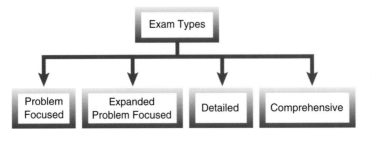

FIGURE 11-2 There are four types of examination: Problem Focused, Expanded Problem Focused, Detailed, and Comprehensive.

TABLE 11.2   Four Types of Examination, as Defined by CPT

Exam Type	CPT Definition
Problem Focused	Limited exam of the problem pertinent body area or organ system
Expanded Problem Focused	Limited exam of the problem pertinent body area or organ system and other related organ system(s)
Detailed	Extended exam of the problem pertinent body area or organ system and other related organ system(s)
Comprehensive	General multisystem exam or complete exam of a single organ system

See CPT E/M Guidelines, "Determine the Extent of Examination Performed"

Comprehensive exam seems to apply only to organ systems and not body areas. Further, how many systems must the physician examine to qualify for a general multisystem exam? Left to define them, different physicians will determine different requirements for the levels. These imprecise definitions are a significant reason why the Centers for Medicare & Medicaid Services (CMS) developed additional guidelines for assigning E&M levels. These guidelines are described in Chapters 14 and 15.

SUMMARY

- The Exam component comprises the objective portion of the SOAP note.
- Exam elements represent the physician's personal observations through inspection, auscultation, palpation, percussion, and other specific testing.
- CPT defines a set of body areas and a set of organ systems in order to determine Exam.
- Do not double-count an exam element by crediting an organ system and a body area for another examination in that organ system.
- Exam will usually be developed using organ systems, except for trauma exams, which may use more appropriate body areas.
- There is no defined endocrine organ system. Thyroid examination is counted under the neck body area.
- Exam may be documented as a narrative or under titles. The titles do not restrict how the comments after the titles are counted.
- There are four types of exam—Problem Focused, Expanded Problem Focused, Detailed, and Comprehensive.
- Exam types are not well defined by CPT.

Chapter Review Exercises

For the following anatomic structures, identify the body area and organ system to which they belong:

1. Brachial artery

2. Appendix

3. Spleen

4. Nose

5. Esophagus

6. Ribs

7. Breast

8. Perineum

9. Thoracic spine

10. Hip joint

CASE STUDY

Revisit the Case Study first presented in Chapter 3. Read the following documentation sample and answer the questions below:

Patient presents with report of foreign object in right eye. Henry Kim is a 35-year-old welder. While at work welding, a metal splinter lodged in his eye.

Exam:

The patient is afebrile and appears in moderate distress, clutching his face. Respirations increased. Heart rate elevated. Patient is slightly diaphoretic. No obvious debris lodged in the face, neck, or hands. Nares clear. Ipsilateral lids normal. Sclera grossly inflamed. Upon examination with slit lamp, the metal splinter is embedded in the cornea but does not enter the anterior chamber. Splinter removed without complication. Contralateral eye is unaffected.

1. Identify the Exam elements in this note by body area.
2. Identify the Exam elements in this note by organ system.
3. Would body areas or organ systems be most appropriate for identifying the Exam elements in this note? Explain.
4. Even though the Exam levels are not well defined, using critical thinking, what level of exam is appropriate? Explain.

12

Medical Decision Making and Assigning an E&M Level

Chapter Outline

I. MDM Component overview

II. Number of Diagnoses or Management Options

III. Amount and/or Complexity of Data to Be Reviewed

IV. Risk of Complications and/or Morbidity or Mortality

V. Four Types of MDM

VI. Assigning an E&M Subcategory Level

LEARNING OUTCOMES

On completion of this chapter, you will be able to:

1. Enumerate the types of Medical Decision Making (MDM).
2. Describe the three elements of MDM.
3. Articulate why additional direction is needed to select an Evaluation and Management (E&M) code objectively.
4. Compile key component data from documentation, and select an E&M level.

KEY TERMS

Diagnosis(es)

Management options

Medical Decision Making (MDM)

Medical Decision Making (MDM) is the third of the three key components required to report component-based Evaluation and Management (E&M) codes. This key component describes the physician's diagnostic assessment and treatment plan for the patient. The diagnostic assessment and treatment plan are expressed in the MDM elements Number of Diagnoses or Management Options, Amount and/or Complexity of Data to Be Reviewed, and Risk of Complications and/or Morbidity or Mortality. The level of documentation of these elements determines which of the three MDM types is correct. This chapter describes MDM as defined by CPT, which differs from the popular Medicare Documentation Guidelines. Additional information on MDM as defined by those Guidelines is included in Chapters 14 and 15.

What part of the SOAP note compares with MDM?

What is the difference between MDM and medical necessity?

What information could be included in the CPT guidelines that would simplify determining MDM?

Including Chapters 10 and 11, are there enough data to assign an E&M level?

MDM COMPONENT OVERVIEW

The final portions of the SOAP note format, Assessment and Plan, correlate with the **Medical Decision Making (MDM)** key component. This component is the least obvious part of an E&M service as it represents the service complexity. MDM attempts to quantify the amount of mental processing the physician employs in developing the patient's diagnosis and treatment plan, which is described by three elements—Number of Diagnoses or Management Options, Amount and/or Complexity of Data to Be Reviewed, and Risk of Complications and/or Morbidity or Mortality (Fig. 12-1).

> **❗ KEY TERM**
>
> Medical Decision Making (MDM)—Key component that describes the Assessment and Plan portions of the visit.

Unfortunately, CPT does not provide much instruction on how to select the correct level of MDM. Although CPT defines levels of each element and four types of MDM, it does not provide guidance on how to arrive at those element levels. The direction provided is even more vague than that provided by CPT for History and Exam. Ultimately, arriving objectively at a type of MDM requires more than using CPT alone.

NUMBER OF DIAGNOSES OR MANAGEMENT OPTIONS

A diagnosis is not the same as a Chief Complaint or presenting problem. Whereas the Chief Complaint is the first building block of an E&M service, the diagnosis is a result of the service. The physician arrives at a **diagnosis** through a process of analysis, considering the patient's History, Exam, other data,

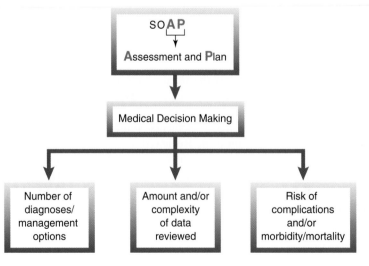

FIGURE 12-1 The final portion of the SOAP note format, Assessment and Plan, correlate with the MDM key component, which is described by 3 elements: Number of Diagnoses or Management Options, Amount and/or Complexity of Data to Be Reviewed, and Risk of Complications and/or Morbidity or Mortality.

Communicating With Medical Providers

Some physicians, in an attempt to quantify the mental diagnostic process, might simply document "moderate level of decision making" and assume that is satisfactory documentation to select moderate complexity of MDM. The coder should discuss with the physician the elements of the MDM component and how they differ from the physician's subjective consideration of the decision-making process. Because what subjectively may be an easy decision for one physician might be more difficult for another physician, MDM attempts to equalize the thought processes by using the disease and treatment documentation as a proxy for the actual cognitive process required to develop a decision.

Having the physician start with an analysis of the complexity of the service provided can assist him or her in documenting an accurate MDM. Encourage the physician to document the mental process step by step—how many diagnoses he/she considered, how much data he/she reviewed, whether he/she spoke to other physicians about the case, how much the patient's condition could affect their life, and so on. Taking the time to describe each step of the decision making process often results in a level of MDM that the physician may have described as "Moderate."

and the physician's knowledge of the condition. Do not confuse the concepts of Chief Complaint and diagnoses. In the SOAP note format, diagnoses are part of the assessment. **Management options** are the plan portion of a SOAP note. Management options include treatment, medications, further testing, requests for consultation by another physician, and any action taken to identify, relieve, or cure the diagnosis.

KEY TERMS

Diagnosis (es)—The underlying cause of symptoms, the nature of an illness.
Management options—Documentation of the plan portion of the visit.

CPT defines four levels of Number of Diagnoses or Management Options—minimal, limited, multiple, and extensive (Fig. 12-2). However, CPT does not provide any guidance on how to distinguish between those levels, and the coder may not infer a level of this element from the physician's general documentation. Therefore, in order to select a level based on CPT directions alone, the physician would have to document the element explicitly — "I considered extensive management options for the patient's diagnosis," which is a rather unusual documentation method.

Following only CPT, a physician could simply state "extensive diagnoses and management options" and appropriately receive the highest element level. This is akin to having the narrative portion of a surgical procedure read "the spleen was removed" without giving any further information. Because payers commonly expect a more complete narrative of the work performed,

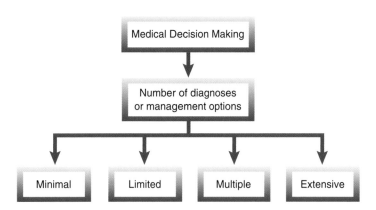

FIGURE 12-2 CPT defines four levels of Number of Diagnoses or Management Options: minimal, limited, multiple, and extensive.

the Medicare Documentation Guidelines provide additional direction on how to select these element levels.

■ AMOUNT AND/OR COMPLEXITY OF DATA TO BE REVIEWED

Although there is no guidance or instruction from CPT, it is assumed that this element refers to diagnostic data. This might include laboratory values, radiological results, invasive diagnostic procedure results, old records, and any other data not received directly from the patient but considered in decision making. CPT describes fours levels for this element—minimal or none, limited, moderate, and extensive (Fig. 12-3). Again, according to CPT, a simple statement from the physician must suffice, "I reviewed a limited amount of data."

■ RISK OF COMPLICATIONS AND/OR MORBIDITY OR MORTALITY

This element, often referred to by the shortened title Risk, has four levels—minimal, low, moderate, and high. The physician should document the risk associated with the patient's Chief Complaint, diagnosis, and/or the management options. The risk can be associated with any or all of these issues, and CPT does not define what constitutes minimal, low, moderate, or high Risk (Fig. 12-4). Following the CPT guidelines, the physician must document the level of risk in that manner, such as "the risk associated with the patient's diagnosis is moderate." In this method, the coder may not infer any level of risk from the physician's documentation; instead this clear risk statement must be documented.

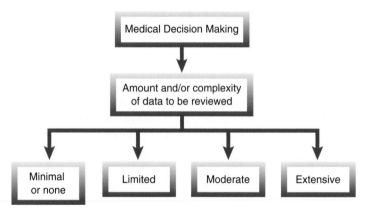

FIGURE 12-3 CPT describes fours levels for the Amount and/or Complexity of Data to be Reviewed element: minimal or none, limited, moderate, and extensive.

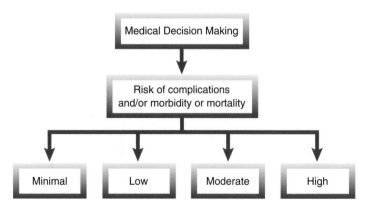

FIGURE 12-4 Risk has four levels—minimal, low, moderate, and high.

■ FOUR TYPES OF MDM

There are four types of MDM—straightforward, low complexity, moderate complexity, and high complexity. Determine the type of MDM based on the levels of the MDM elements. Table 12.1 describes the four MDM types and their related element levels.

Take note that MDM differs from History when determining the component type. History requires that the minimum level for all three elements be met in order to report the History type. However, MDM only requires that *any two* of the three element levels be met in order to report the MDM type. A common misconception is that the MDM type cannot be higher than the Risk will allow. However, all three elements have equal weight, and any two of the three can be used to select the MDM type.

CRITICAL THINKING

It could make sense that the Risk element should have more weight in determining the MDM type, but why are all of the elements considered with the same weight? When would one of the other two elements have more weight than Risk?

■ Example of typical MDM

Considering the sample patient from Chapters 10 and 11 who presented with a sore throat, typical MDM might be documented as, "Rapid strep positive. Prescribed Amoxicillin t.i.d. 10 days for strep throat. Continue warm salt-water gargle as tolerated. Soft food and ample fluids, slowly reintroduce solid foods. Return to school when fever is resolved and patient is not fatigued."

According to CPT guidelines, the coder cannot determine an MDM type from this note. The physician would need to include atypical notes such as, "Diagnosis with minimal risk of complications, multiple management options, and limited data reviewed." Because there are no guidelines to define these element levels, assume the physician's notes are correct. Table 12.2 summarizes the MDM elements for the sample patient.

Because only two of the three element minimums must be met, start by excluding the lowest element level. Then, select the MDM based on the lowest level element documented. Risk of Complications and/or Morbidity or Mortality has the lowest element level, so exclude it from consideration. Whereas Number of Diagnoses and/or Treatment Options is documented as Multiple ("multiple management

TABLE 12.1   MDM Types and Element Minimums* for Each Type

MDM Type	Number of Diagnoses and/or Treatment Options	Amount and/or Complexity of Data to Be Reviewed	Risk of Complications and/or Morbidity or Mortality
Straightforward	Minimal	Minimal or None	Minimal
Low Complexity	Limited	Limited	Low
Moderate Complexity	Multiple	Moderate	Moderate
High Complexity	Extensive	Extensive	High

*2 of the 3 element minimums must be met.

TABLE 12.2 Summary MDM for Sample Patient

MDM Type	Number of Diagnoses and/or Treatment Options	Amount and/or Complexity of Data to Be Reviewed	Risk of Complications and/or Morbidity or Mortality
Straightforward	Minimal	Minimal or None	**Minimal**
Low Complexity	Limited	**Limited**	Low
Moderate Complexity	**Multiple**	Moderate	Moderate
High Complexity	Extensive	Extensive	High

options"), Amount and/or Complexity of Data to Be Reviewed is documented as "limited data reviewed" and has the lowest remaining element level, so the MDM type is Low Complexity. Another way to consider how to select the MDM type is by choosing the type that corresponds to the middle element level.

ASSIGNING AN E&M SUBCATEGORY LEVEL

Using the information from Chapters 10, 11, and 12, a component-based E&M service code can be assigned. The HPI note in Chapter 10 describes the patient as "well-known to the practice." For the purposes of this example, assume the patient visit is with his pediatrician in an outpatient office setting. The correct E&M category for the visit is Office or Other Outpatient Services (99201–99205, 99211–99215). Also assume that, as the patient is described as well known to the practice, his pediatrician has seen him within the last 3 years, making this is an Established Patient (99211–99215). A summary of the patient's visit is included in Table 12.3. Finally, for the purposes of the example, assume the Exam is Problem Focused.

To select an E&M level, the key component minimums must be met for either 2 of 3 or 3 of 3 key components, according to the E&M code description. Office or Other Outpatient Services, Established Patient levels require only 2 of 3 key component minimums. For codes that require only 2 of 3 key component minimums, disregard the lowest component type, and then select the E&M level with the next lowest component type. Put another way, select the E&M level corresponding to the middle component type. In the example in Table 12.3, disregard the Exam because it is the lowest component type, and select the E&M level based on the next lowest component type, MDM, which results in selecting 99213. Similar to MDM and Risk, a misconception regarding codes that require 2 of 3 key components minimums be met is that the level cannot be higher than the corresponding MDM type. Again, all 3 components have equal weight, and any 2 of the 3 can be used to select the E&M level. At the beginning of the E&M chapter in the CPT manual, there is a complete summary of component-based E&M codes with grids similar to Table 12.3 of the required minimum key components.

TABLE 12.3 Summary of Sample Patient Visit Documentation From Chapters 10–12

E/M Subcategory Level	History (Chapter 10)	Exam (Chapter 11)	MDM (Chapter 12)	Meet Requirements? (At least 2 of the 3 key component minimums are met.)
99211	Does not require the presence of a physician.			Yes
99212	Problem focused	**Problem Focused**	Straightforward	Yes
99213	Expanded Problem Focused	Expanded Problem Focused	**Low**	**Yes**
99214	**Detailed**	Detailed	Moderate	No
99215	Comprehensive	Comprehensive	High	No

● ● ● SUMMARY

- The MDM component comprises the Assessment and Plan portions of a SOAP format note.
- MDM represents the mental process of arriving at a diagnosis and treating the patient's condition.
- The three elements of MDM are Number of Diagnoses or Management Options, Amount and/or Complexity of Data to Be Reviewed, and Risk of Complications and/or Morbidity or Mortality.
- The four MDM types are straightforward, low complexity, moderate complexity, and high complexity.
- Only 2 of the 3 element levels must be met to select an MDM type.
- All 3 elements have equal weight in determining the MDM type.
- All 3 key components have equal weight in determining the E&M level.
- The highest E&M level at which all of the required component type minimums are met is the correct E&M level.

Chapter Review Exercises

Using Table 12.1 as a guide, select the correct MDM type based on the listed information.

Question	Number of Diagnoses and/or Treatment Options	Amount and/or Complexity of Data to Be Reviewed	Risk of Complications and/or Morbidity or Mortality	MDM Type
1.	Limited	Moderate	High	
2.	Multiple	Limited	Minimal	
3.	Extensive	Extensive	Low	
4.	Multiple	Minimal	High	
5.	Minimal	Minimal	Moderate	

For the following questions, note whether the code requires 2 of 3 or 3of 3 key component minimums, and select the correct E&M level. Refer to the tables in CPT as a guide.

Question	Category	Subcategory	History	Exam	MDM	2 of 3 or 3 of 3	E&M Level
6.	Office or Other Outpatient Services	New	Detailed	Detailed	Low Complexity		
7.	Office or Other Outpatient Services	Established	Detailed	Detailed	Low Complexity		
8.	Emergency	N/A	Detailed	Detailed	Low Complexity		
9.	Hospital Inpatient Services	Initial Hospital Care	Comprehensive	Comprehensive	High Complexity		
10.	Hospital Inpatient Services	Subsequent Hospital Care	Detailed	Problem focused	Moderate Complexity		

CASE STUDIES

Case Study 1

Revisit the Case Study first presented in Chapter 3. Read the following documentation sample, and answer the questions below:

[Patient presents with report of foreign object in right eye. Henry Kim is a 35-year-old welder. While at work welding, a metal splinter lodged in his eye.]

MDM:

Under slit lamp examination, metal splinter is visualized embedded in cornea at 5 o'clock position. Splinter was removed without complication. Usual bandaging was applied, and the patient was sent home with instructions to keep the bandage dry and in place for 3 days. Patient instructed to follow-up with Dr. Wheaton, ophthalmologist, or return to the ED, if vision does not improve or any new symptoms occur. I considered multiple diagnoses and treatment options and did not review any additional data. There is moderate risk of loss of vision or other damage to the eye from this condition.

1. Identify the level of Number of Diagnoses or Management Options.
2. Identify the level of Amount and/or Complexity of Data to Be Reviewed.
3. Identify the level of Risk of Complication and/or Morbidity or Mortality.
4. Identify the element at the lowest level.
5. Determine the MDM type.

Case Study 2

Review the case studies from Chapters 10, 11, and 12 in total as the documentation for an E&M visit.

1. Select the E&M Category
2. Select the Subcategory, if applicable
3. Does the code series require 2 of 3 or 3 of 3 key component minimums to be met?
4. Determine the correct E&M Level for the visit.

Case Study 3

In the Chapter 9 Case Study, Mr. Kim saw Dr. Bellkey because of his borderline blood glucose levels. Read the following sample documentation. Using the information presented in Chapters 4–12, answer the questions below.

[This is the first time Mr. Kim has seen Dr. Bellkey. He goes to see her in her office in a downtown medical building.]

Mr. Kim is a 35-year-old welder by trade who was found to have borderline glucose levels during a hospital stay 1 month ago. The levels were higher after meals but never exceeded 200 mg/dL. The patient thinks he might have experienced some frequent urination, but that could be from increased fluid intake. Since his hospital stay, the patient has been concerned about his blood sugar and has started walking 20 minutes at least 5 days/week, and reducing his caloric intake.

Mr. Kim reports no recent weight changes or changes in appetite. His vision has returned to normal since his corneal transplant. He has not noticed any recent cuts or bruises that are slow to heal. No extremity tingling or numbness. No oral infections. No skin infections. No bladder infections. Normal bowel movements. No shortness of breath, no chest pains.

Continued

CASE STUDIES—cont'd

Patient reports his knees hurt from time to time from remote history of athletics, but pain is controlled with ibuprofen. No depression, slight anxiety concerning healing eye trauma. No other current endocrine symptoms or disease. Patient is immunosuppressed due to the corneal transplant and reports his medication is preventing rejection.

No other medications. Patient reports paternal grandfather developed type II diabetes over 60. No other diabetic history. Patient is a welder and has recently started an exercise routine.

Exam:

Head: normocephalic, atraumatic

Neck: supple, trachea midline, no lymphadenopathy

Eyes: grossly normal

ENMT: mucous membranes pink

Cardiovascular: RRR

Respiratory: clear breath sounds bilateral

GI: Postive bowel sounds, no organomegaly

GU: external genitalia normal, no hernias palpated

Extremities: full ROM in all four extremities; positive reflexes and strength ×4; no skin changes noted

Neuro: cranial nerves II–XII normal; patient is oriented ×3

Data Reviewed:

Patient had a fasting blood sugar 3 days ago 90 mg/dL, which is high normal.

Cholesterol also elevated but WNL.

Other labs were normal.

Assessment and Plan:

Mr. Kim had recent elevated blood sugars, but latest test shows high normal. At this time I would not consider him diabetic or prediabetic, given his absence of symptoms and transient blood sugar levels. Mr. Kim should continue new diet and exercise habits. I gave him a pamphlet today on healthy eating. Mr. Kim should see me every 6 months to monitor his progress and hopefully avoid any disease process. Should his blood sugars start to increase, we will revisit his diagnosis and treatment. I considered multiple treatment options and reviewed a moderate amount of data. At this point, I think Mr. Kim has a moderate risk of developing type II diabetes at some point in the future.

Identify the following information about this E&M service, or answer the question:
1. Category
2. Subcategory
3. Chief Complaint
4. Elements of HPI
5. HPI level (For this exercise, consider 1–3 elements = Brief, 4–7 elements = Extended.)
6. Systems of review
7. Problem pertinent system
8. ROS level
9. Elements of PFSH
10. PFSH level
11. History type
12. Exam elements in this note by body area
13. Exam elements in this note by organ system
14. Would body areas or organ systems be most appropriate for identifying the Exam elements in this note? Explain.

CASE STUDIES—cont'd

15. Even though the Exam levels are not well defined, using critical thinking, what level of Exam is appropriate? Explain.
16. Number of Diagnoses or Management Options level
17. Amount and/or Complexity of Data to Be Reviewed level
18. Risk of Complication and/or Morbidity or Mortality level
19. Lowest level of MDM
20. MDM type
21. Does this code series require 2 of 3 or 3 of 3 key component minimums to be met?
22. Restate the History, Exam, and MDM levels
23. What E&M code should be reported for this visit?

Contributing Components and Time

Chapter Outline

I. Counseling and Coordination of Care

II. Nature of Presenting Problem

III. Time

IV. Time as the Principal Component

LEARNING OUTCOMES

On completion of this chapter, you will be able to:

1. Identify the three contributing Evaluation and Management (E&M) components.
2. Identify the seventh E&M component.
3. Articulate how Nature of Presenting Problem can affect the E&M level.
4. Define intraservice time in office and hospital settings.
5. Use time-based E&M level selection as an alternative to key components.

KEY TERMS

Coordination of Care	Intraservice time	Principal component
Counseling	Nature of Presenting	
Face-to-face	Problem (NOPP)	

Although there is considerable focus in E&M coding on the three key components, there are four additional components to an E&M service—three contributing components and the component of Time. The three contributing components are Counseling, Coordination of Care, and Nature of Presenting Problem (Fig. 13-1). This chapter focuses on situations when, instead of the key components, Counseling and Coordination of Care dominate a visit, and Time becomes the key, or principal, component.

Focus Questions

How does the Nature of Presenting Problem affect E&M levels?

Why is intraservice time measured differently in the office than in the hospital?

How much time must be spent in Counseling and/or Coordination of Care to use time-based coding?

What are the three elements of time-based coding?

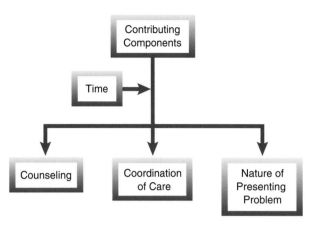

FIGURE 13-1 There are four additional components to an E&M service: Time, Counseling, Coordination of Care, and Nature of Presenting Problem.

■ COUNSELING AND COORDINATION OF CARE

Counseling and Coordination of Care are two of the three contributing components to an E&M level and are often addressed in tandem. **Counseling** consists of the physician's discussion with the patient and the patient's family and/or the patient's decision maker regarding diagnosis and treatment options. It is essentially discussing the Assessment and Plan portions of the SOAP note and answering any of the patient's questions. **Coordination of Care** includes writing prescriptions, ordering diagnostic tests, deciding to request consultations, scheduling procedures, and coordinating other services that will occur later that are associated with the visit (Fig. 13-2).

> **❗ KEY TERMS**
>
> Counseling—Contributing component that describes the physician discussing diagnosis and treatment options with the patient.
> Coordination of Care—Contributing component that includes ordering diagnostic studies, planning return visits, asking a nurse to complete incidental care, and other associated services.

Counseling and Coordination of Care do not need to occur at every visit and will not necessarily be documented (see Fig. 13-2). Documented or not, they do not affect the E&M level selected for a key component–based service when key components comprise the majority of the service,

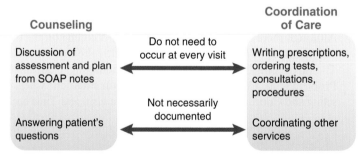

FIGURE 13-2 Counseling and Coordination of Care are two of the three contributing components to an E&M level and are often addressed in tandem. Counseling consists of the physician's discussion with the patient and the patient's family and/or the patient's decision maker regarding diagnosis and treatment options. Coordination of Care includes writing prescriptions, ordering diagnostic tests, deciding to request consultations, scheduling procedures, and coordinating other services that will occur later that are associated with the visit.

which is why they are called contributing components. However, it is good practice to document all services performed during the visit and all planned services in order to have a complete record of the visit.

CRITICAL THINKING

Why are Counseling and Coordination of Care not considered key components?

◼ NATURE OF PRESENTING PROBLEM

Unlike Counseling and Coordination of Care, the third contributing component, **Nature of Presenting Problem (NOPP),** can affect the E&M level. NOPP describes the potential severity of the patient's Chief Complaint. It provides subjective information that might be used to determine the appropriate E&M level. CPT describes five levels of NOPP—minimal, self-limited or minor, low severity, moderate severity, and high severity (Fig. 13-3). Each key component–based E&M code includes information about the general level of NOPP for which a physician would perform that level of service. For example, the code description for Office or Other Outpatient Services, New Patient, 99203, states that the presenting problem usually is of moderate severity. Each key component–based code description includes this guidance in the last paragraph of the description.

❗ KEY TERMS

Nature of Presenting Problem (NOPP)—Contributing component that is much more of a conceptual component, describing how many differential diagnoses a presenting problem creates, or the typical outcome for a presenting problem.

When the NOPP level is significantly lower than the documented key components, the coder might consider whether the key components as documented were medically necessary based on the Chief Complaint. A classic example is a patient who presents to the Emergency Department (ED) with upper respiratory symptoms. The attending physician completes a full work-up according to ED protocol and determines the patient probably has a common cold virus but prescribes an antibiotic as a cautionary measure. The physician could accurately document the key components for the visit as a 99284. However, note in the CPT manual the NOPP level for 99284 is high severity, which is much higher than the patient's presenting problem would suggest. After discussion with the physician, the E&M level might be reduced to 99283. This is a subjective decision that only experienced coders should make, and they will often make it with agreement from the treating physician, another coder, or supervisor.

Novice coders will sometimes confuse NOPP and Medical Decision Making (MDM) and follow the misconception that an E&M level higher than the MDM type allows can never be assigned. This is not correct, and coders should be careful not to confuse the two concepts. As a key component, MDM has equal weight with History and Exam. NOPP should be used as a reducing factor only occasionally and with caution.

FIGURE 13-3 The third contributing component, Nature of Presenting Problem (NOPP), could affect the E&M level. CPT describes five levels of NOPP: minimal, self-limited or minor, low severity, moderate severity, and high severity.

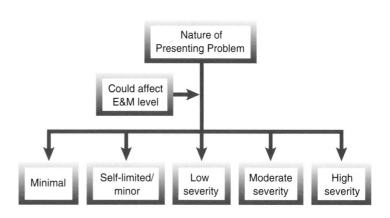

■ TIME

The seventh component of most E&M codes is Time. In some instances, codes are inherently time-based and are always coded based on the specific time a physician expends. CPT considers time to be a significant factor in assisting with selecting the correct code, which may explain some of the vague direction given for key components. CPT includes in the E&M section guidelines that time is a proxy for effort in assigning E&M levels. CPT intends for the listed times in E&M codes to be an average of **intraservice time** spent during an E&M service (Fig. 13-4). In practice, most payers consider the times in key component–based codes as a minimum requirement for reporting the code.

❗ KEY TERMS

Intraservice time—Time spent face-to-face with the patient.

CPT defines intraservice time differently depending on the place of service. In the office and other outpatient settings, intraservice time refers to time the physician spends **face-to-face** with the patient, literally in the presence of the patient (see Fig. 13-4). Review the code description in the CPT manual for Office or Other Outpatient Services, Established Patient, 99214. This code description states the physician usually spends about 25 minutes face-to-face with a patient. The physician might spend this time discussing the patient's diagnosis and treatment options. The physician might also review test results, discuss the case with another provider, or take other actions not directly involving the patient, but the activities must be completed in the presence of the patient to credit the time toward the service.

❗ KEY TERMS

Face-to-face—Working in the physical presence of the patient. For hospital visits, also time spent on the unit/floor dedicated to the patient.

In the hospital and other inpatient settings, intraservice time is both time spent face-to-face with the patient and time spent on the patient's floor or unit that is devoted to that patient (see Fig. 13-4). The difference is based on practice. In the office, usually the preponderance of the visit is in the exam room with the patient. Certainly, some other work, especially coordination of care, might be done without the patient, but it is considered too small and too varied to be measured with consistency. In the hospital, a physician will probably do a significant amount of work outside of a patient's room but while

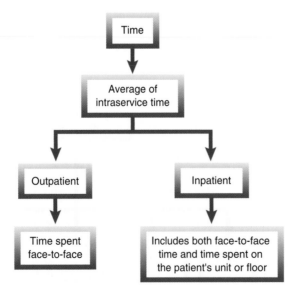

FIGURE 13-4 The seventh component of most E&M codes is Time. CPT intends for the listed times in E&M codes to be an average of intraservice time spent during an E&M service.

still on the patient's floor. For example, if a physician spends 70 minutes admitting a patient, discussing the treatment plan with the patient and family, reviewing lab and radiology results at the nurses' station, and discussing a consultation with another physician on the patient's unit, the appropriate code to report is 99223, Initial Hospital Care.

 CRITICAL THINKING

Why do Emergency Department Services not include average intraservice time?

TIME AS THE PRINCIPAL COMPONENT

When Counseling and Coordination of Care comprise a majority of an otherwise key component–based service, then Time becomes the **principal component.** The CPT manual E&M section guidelines dictate the physician must document the total intraservice time spent and that more than 50% of the visit was spent in Counseling and/or Coordination of Care. The documentation can be worded in many ways, as long as it is clear that more than half the time was spent on these activities.

KEY TERMS

Principal component—Time becomes the overwhelming factor for the visit when Counseling and Coordination of Care comprise the majority of the visit

Examples of majority statements

- "More than half the visit was spent in counseling and coordination of care."
- "We spent most of the visit discussing…"
- "More than 50% of the visit…"
- "25 of 30 minutes focused on discussing…"
- "The entire visit comprised…"

The physician must also document a summary of the discussion and may or may not perform key components during the visit. Key components are not required, and they do not affect the E&M level. Compare the following note with the previous chapter examples of the visit for the 10-year-old patient with a sore throat.

Example of Time as the principal component

The patient is an otherwise healthy 10-year-old boy, well known to the practice, who presents with a history of increasingly sore throat and difficulty swallowing. This is the patient's fourth visit in 6 months with similar symptoms. On exam the throat is red and swollen, with signs of chronic inflammation. Rapid strep was positive. I spent almost the entire visit discussing chronic strep throat infections with the patient's mother and whether surgical intervention was appropriate. It is my opinion that the infections are occurring with significant frequency, and a tonsillectomy is warranted. The patient's mother agreed, and I gave her an ENT referral. I spent a total of 25 minutes with the patient and his mother.

The physician does take some history, performs an exam, and reviews the rapid strep test but spends the majority of the visit in counseling with the mother, discussing the patient's diagnosis and how best to treat the patient. The conversation probably included discussing the different treatment options, indicating why the physician thought surgery was best, and answering the mother's questions about the procedure and typical recovery. The physician documented the total intraservice time, specified that a majority of the time was spent counseling, and included a summary of the discussion, so the key components are not a factor in determining the E&M level for this visit. Instead, Time is the principal component. For an established patient, this 25-minute visit can be reported with 99214. Based on the key components alone, the visit would be at best 99213, perhaps only 99212.

CRITICAL THINKING

Based on the preceding note, if the visit were coded based on key components, would you select 99212 or 99213? Why?

Communicating With Medical Providers

Physicians are often surprised that the time-based coding documentation requirements are seemingly lower than those for key component–based coding for the same visit. Some physicians will not remember that when using time-based coding the majority of the visit must be spent in Counseling and Coordination of Care and may not be used when key components dominate the visit. Always be clear about the requirements for Time-based coding. The visit is either coded with key components or based on Time, but not both. There is also not a choice between coding based on key components or Time. If the visit meets the criteria for Time-based coding, Time must be used as the principal component.

SUMMARY

- Counseling and Coordination of Care are contributing components that the physician does not have to document for every visit.
- Nature of Presenting Problem (NOPP) is a contributing component that experienced coders may use to gauge the appropriate E&M level.
- Time is the seventh component.
- According to CPT, the listed time in E&M codes are averages, not minimums, but common practice describes them as minimums.
- Office and other outpatient service intraservice time is time spent face-to-face with the patient.
- Hospital and other inpatient service intraservice time is time spent face-to-face with patients and also time spent devoted to patients on their floor or unit.
- When a majority of the visit is spent in Counseling and/or Coordination of Care, Time is the principal component.
- If a visit meets the criteria for time-based coding, key component–based coding may not be used.
- For time-based coding, the physician must document the total intraservice time, specify that a majority of the time was spent in Counseling and/or Coordination of Care, and include a summary of the discussion.

Chapter Review Exercises

1. What is the average intraservice time for a consultation provided in an inpatient setting that includes a documented comprehensive history, detailed exam, and medical decision making of moderate complexity?

2. What is the average intraservice time for an initial visit in a skilled nursing facility that includes a documented comprehensive history, comprehensive exam, and medical decision making of low complexity?

Assign the correct E&M code using time-based coding for the following note excerpts:

3. A 50-year-old patient who has not been seen before in the practice is seen by an internist in the office to discuss his anxiety and management options. A majority of the visit is spent in counseling. The visit lasts 20 minutes.

4. A cardiac surgeon sees an existing patient in the office to discuss the patient's diagnosis of valve stenosis and management options. They spend 40 minutes together, discussing the risks of surgery versus waiting for symptoms to develop further and possible mortality associated with both options.

5. A hospitalist admits an 85-year-old patient with adult failure to thrive. The hospitalist spends 50 minutes with the patient, all of which is spent discussing the underlying possibilities of the diagnosis and the patient's desired outcomes.

6. An endocrinologist, who previously admitted the patient, talks with a patient on hospital day 3, primarily discussing whether to continue with medical management or to make a referral for surgery. The visit lasts 15 minutes.

7. A gerontologist makes a scheduled visit to a patient's home; during the visit they spend 25 minutes discussing the patient's multiple diagnoses and whether the patient should be admitted or continue to be monitored at home.

In order to code based on Time, describe what is missing in the following note excerpts:

8. I spent the entire visit discussing the management options for scoliosis with the patient and her mother. The patient had many questions about bracing and possible surgical correction. As the patient is in her teens, she also expressed considerable social anxiety.

9. Patient presents with intermittent gross hematuria × 2 weeks. A comprehensive history was obtained. On examination, vital signs within normal limits. The external genitalia are normal, no hernias or enlarged lymph nodes can be palpated. RRR, bilateral breath sounds.
   I spent 20 minutes with the patient, a majority of which was in counseling and coordination of care.

10. The patient and her father presented again today with the complaint that the child is fussy, has again had a fever, and is pulling at her ears. Presumed recurrent otitis media. I talked with the father about bilateral tympanoplasty. Total visit time was 15 minutes.

CASE STUDY

Consider Mr. Kim's visits below. Assign the correct E&M code for each encounter using time-based coding. Assume that all services are documented and meet the requirements for time-based coding.

[Mr. Kim, a welder, was first seen in the Emergency Department for a metal splinter lodged in his eye.]

As the next few weeks went by, Henry's vision became increasingly blurry, his eye watered continuously, and he continued to experience pain. Henry went to a local ophthalmologist, Dr. Wheaton, for further treatment and was new to the practice. Dr. Wheaton determined that the emergency physician did not remove the entire metal splinter from Henry's cornea. It was the ophthalmologist's opinion that the cornea had been permanently scarred, and the only treatment that would restore Henry's vision would be a corneal transplant. Dr. Wheaton spent a majority of the visit, which lasted a total of 20 minutes, discussing corneal transplant with Mr. Kim.

1. Select the E&M code for Dr. Wheaton's visit.

Because corneal transplants are an expensive treatment, Henry's Workers Compensation insurance carrier wanted him to have a second opinion from Dr. Samson, an ophthalmologist, who also happened to perform corneal transplants at the academic medical center in Omaha, Nebraska. Henry traveled to Omaha, about 3 hours away, to see the second ophthalmologist, who agreed that a transplant was necessary. Henry was also new to Dr. Samson's practice. Dr. Samson agreed with Dr. Wheaton's assessment of Henry's condition and discussed the associated risks and considerations of corneal transplant and the process to become a candidate for transplant with the patient for 25 of a 30-minute visit.

2. Select the E&M code for Dr. Samson's visit.

Henry had surgery, and the transplant was a success. During his preoperative workup, Henry was found to have borderline glucose levels. Dr. Samson asked an endocrinologist, Dr. Lester, to evaluate Henry for diabetes while he was inpatient. Dr. Lester saw Henry bedside and completed his note in the shared medical record. Dr. Lester determined that Henry did not have diabetes but should be monitored regularly when he returned home. They also discussed some recommendations about diet and exercise. More than 50% of Dr. Lester's visit was spent counseling the patient. Dr. Lester spent 10 minutes face-to-face with the patient and 10 minutes at the nurses' station reviewing labs and other notes for the case. Henry was discharged home after 2 days.

CASE STUDY—cont'd

3. Select the E&M code for Dr. Lester's visit.

About 6 months after surgery, Henry saw an endocrinologist in Grand Island, Dr. Bellkey, as a new patient for a recheck of his glucose levels. Dr. Bellkey spent most of the visit counseling Henry on the risks of diabetes and the importance of diet and exercise. Dr. Bellkey thought Henry was doing well and asked him to return in a year for a recheck. They spent a total of 45 minutes face-to-face. Before Henry arrived, Dr. Bellkey also spent 15 minutes in her office reviewing his blood sugars over time, additional laboratory results, and his inpatient notes.

4. Select the E&M code for Dr. Bellkey's visit.

Medicare Evaluation and Management Guidelines

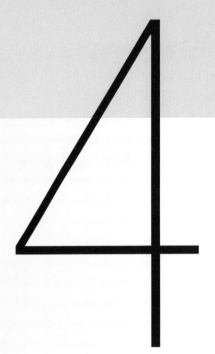

14

Medicare 1995 Documentation Guidelines

Chapter Outline

LEARNING OUTCOMES

On completion of this chapter, you will be able to:

1. Assign an Evaluation and Management (E&M) service level using the Medicare 1995 Documentation Guidelines.
2. Distinguish the differences between CPT and Medicare documentation guidelines.
3. Use an audit tool to assign an E&M service level.

KEY TERMS

All Others Negative (AON)	Qualitative	ROS–Extended
Duration	Quantitative	ROS–N/A
HPI–Brief	PFSH–Complete	ROS–Problem Pertinent
HPI–Extended	PFSH–Pertinent	
Legible	ROS–Complete	

As described in the preceding chapters, the CPT E&M guidelines describe service levels in **qualitative** terms. The Medicare 1995 Documentation Guidelines (1995 Guidelines) attempt to describe service levels in a more **quantitative** manner. This chapter describes how to assign an E&M service level based on the 1995 Guidelines. The chapter also describes the differences between the two sets of guidelines and where the 1995 Guidelines are still qualitative instead of quantitative.

Focus Questions

What documentation element must be present in every E&M note?

What are the two elements of an E&M note that do not need to be documented by the billing physician?

What portions of the Medicare 1995 Documentation Guidelines are vague?

❗ KEY TERMS

Qualitative—Measured by descriptive terms.
Quantitative—Measured by the amount of information documented.

■ MEDICARE 1995 DOCUMENTATION GUIDELINES

After the AMA developed new E&M Guidelines for CPT in 1992, Medicare found those guidelines could be applied too variably. Because Medicare fee-for-service reimburses a set rate for any E&M code, the service represented by a code needed to be consistent. The CPT E&M guidelines were too qualitative to provide for a consistent service level. What one physician practice considered a brief History of Present Illness (HPI) could be considered extensive by another practice. Medicare reviewers were not able to apply a consistent methodology in determining whether the reported code appropriately represented the service rendered. Thus, Medicare leadership developed a more quantitative method of determining E&M service levels. However, translating E&M notes into completely quantitative terms eludes the industry to the current day. The 1995 Guidelines, while quantifying many aspects of the E&M service, left some areas open to interpretation.

For example, the opening paragraphs of the 1995 Guidelines note that E&M services for infants, children, adolescents, and pregnant women might not follow the guidelines since care for these populations varies considerably from the service generally provided to an adult patient. For these special populations, the 1995 Guidelines do not provide specific, complete guidance as to what would be an appropriate note to support reporting any specific code. In practice, reviewers typically follow the guidelines as much as possible for these patients, but subjective judgments need to be made when the documentation does not correlate the typical note to support a code.

Conversely, the 1995 Guidelines did define some fundamental guidelines now widely used for all E&M services. They are so fundamental to documentation standards that many reviewers do not realize they are part of any official guidelines. These guidelines include that the documented note for the service must support all E&M codes reported to Medicare. The documentation is considered the complete record of the service and must be **legible.** The industry standard for note legibility is if three trained reviewers are unable to read the note, it is not legible. The physician must also sign the note legibly and date the note. Signature legibility can include that a reviewer can match the signature to a signature log. It is critical to read the 1995 Guidelines (see Medicare 1995 Documentation Guidelines in Appendix A) in their entirety, to read them along with this text, and to reread them occasionally throughout one's career. Many coders forget some of the lesser-used rules or diverge from a requirement without realizing it.

❗ KEY TERMS

Legible—As least one of three reviewers must be able to read the note.

◼ HISTORY

Another fundamental guideline is that the billing physician must personally document the entire note, except for Review of Systems (ROS) and Past, Family, Social History (PFSH), which can be documented by the patient, a medical assistant, or any other personnel. If the billing physician does not personally document ROS and PFSH, the physician must reference those elements with the date and location of the elements in the record. If the elements were documented on another day, the physician must note whether there are any updates necessary. It is important to note these are the only two elements specifically described in the 1995 Guidelines the billing physician need not document personally. The physician must document the Chief Complaint and History of Present Illness (HPI) personally.

The 1995 Guidelines clearly define how many elements of History the physician must document to achieve each level of History. Except for the new component quantification, the CPT guidelines still apply. The minimum element levels must be met in order to select a History type. The coder selects the History based on the lowest level element documented. Because the code selection is based on evidence of physician effort, not the patient's answers, both positive and negative answers count toward the code.

The 1995 Guidelines, as in CPT guidelines, define two types of HPI—Brief and Extended. However, unlike CPT, 1995 Guidelines define **HPI—Brief** as 1–3 documented elements and **HPI—Extended** as 4 or more elements. The 1995 Guidelines also add an eighth History of Present Illness (HPI) element not included in CPT—**Duration** (Fig. 14-1). The difference between Duration and Timing is that Duration describes how long the Chief Complaint has existed, and Timing describes some pattern by which the Chief Complaint occurs. For example, the Chief Complaint may have begun 1 week ago (duration) and is worse in the morning (timing). Table 14.1 includes the description of the eight elements recognized in the 1995 Guidelines.

❗ KEY TERMS

HPI–Brief—1 to 3 elements of HPI
HPI–Extended—4 or more elements of HPI
Duration—How long the patient has had the Chief Complaint

◼ Example of an Extended HPI

In the HPI of the patient first presented in Chapter 10, there are more than 4 HPI elements documented, so the HPI is Extended.

HPI: The patient is an otherwise healthy 10-year-old boy, well known to the practice, who presents with a history of increasingly sore throat and difficulty swallowing. He describes the soreness as scratchy and feels it is worse in the morning. He has tried gargling warm salt water with little effect. His mother reports he has also had a low-grade fever for 2 days. There have been children in his class out sick with strep throat in recent weeks.

Chief Complaint: sore throat
Elements:
Location—throat
Quality—scratchy
Severity—increasingly
Timing—worse in the morning
Context—schoolmates recently sick with strep throat
Modifying factors—gargling warm salt water
Associated signs & symptoms—difficulty swallowing, low-grade fever

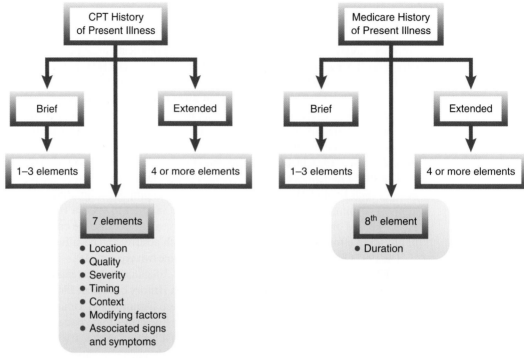

FIGURE 14-1 Elements of History of Present Illness.

TABLE 14.1 HPI Elements, Including Duration

Element	Definition	Examples
Location	Anatomical body part	Right leg Throat LUQ All over Abdomen
Quality	How the patient characterizes the Chief Complaint (usually an adjective for the Chief Complaint)	Sharp, dull, throbbing, or radiating (pain) Persistent Dry/wet (cough)
Severity	How bad, or how difficult it is to endure, the Chief Complaint	Pain on a scale Worse than... Mild, moderate, severe Better/worse So bad that is causes some effect
Duration	How long the patient has had the Chief Complaint	Two months A few weeks Since childhood
Timing	Frequency of the Chief Complaint, or patterns in when the Chief Complaint occurs	Every morning All the time Intermittent Usually in the evening
Context	Conditions that cause the Chief Complaint to occur Conditions present in the patient's environment when it occurs	When the patient stands up The patient fell When the patient pets her dog If the patient runs more than 20 minutes Only when the patient is sleeping

TABLE 14.1 HPI Elements, Including Duration—cont'd

Element	Definition	Examples
Modifying Factors	What the patient has done to try and resolve the problem	Ice and ibuprofen Takes as many as 6 antacid tablets 3×day Stretches when standing Better after 30 minutes rest Has not tried anything
Associated Signs & Symptoms	Other conditions that occur with the Chief Complaint	Nausea & vomiting Pain Blurred vision Numbness No other complaints

ROS is categorized by four types in 1995 Guidelines—**N/A**, **Problem Pertinent**, **Extended**, and **Complete**. These types are defined in Table 14.2.

! KEY TERMS

ROS–Problem Pertinent—1 system reviewed
ROS–Extended—2 to 9 systems reviewed
ROS–Complete—10 to 14 systems reviewed

▌ Example of an Extended ROS

In the ROS of the patient first presented in Chapter 10, there are 9 systems reviewed, so the ROS is Extended.

ROS: The patient has been sleeping well and has not had any recent weight loss. No report of itching eyes. His nose has started to run today. CV negative. His mother says his breathing has not been labored. No achiness. No rashes. The patient has mild environmental allergies and has not recently been exposed to any new allergens.

Constitutional—sleeping well; no recent weight loss
Eyes—no report of itching eyes
ENMT—runny nose
Cardiovascular—negative
Respiratory—breathing is not labored
Musculoskeletal—no achiness
Integumentary—no rashes
Allergic/immunological—mild environmental allergies

TABLE 14.2 1995 Guidelines Review of Systems Types and Element Minimums

ROS Type	N/A	Problem Pertinent	Extended	Complete
Element minimum	None	1 problem pertinent system	Problem pertinent system, and 1–8 additional systems (2–9 systems total)	Problem pertinent system, and 9–13 additional systems (10–14 systems total)

The 1995 Guidelines also allow a summary method of documenting ROS—Complete. If all 14 systems are reviewed, the problem pertinent system is documented, any positive systems are documented, and any pertinent negative systems are documented, then the physician can abbreviate the remaining systems by documenting, **"all others negative (AON)"** (Fig. 14-2). The rules for this shortcut are very specific and must be performed in this way. Review the 1995 Guidelines ROS section, and note this permitted exception.

❗ KEY TERMS

All Others Negative (AON)—An abbreviation used to indicate all systems were reviewed and the non-problem pertinent systems were negative.

The 1995 Guidelines define two types of **PFSH—Pertinent** and **Complete.** PFSH—Pertinent requires documentation of 1 element of 1 history. PFSH—Complete requires documentation of 1 element of 2 or 3 histories, depending on the E&M service type, listed in Table 14.3. Note that, according to the 1995 Guidelines, PSFH is not a required element for Subsequent Hospital Care (99231–99233), Subsequent Observation Care (99224–99226), and Subsequent Nursing Facility Care (99307–99310).

❗ KEY TERMS

PFSH–Pertinent—1 History type, past, family or social
PFSH–Complete—2 or 3 History types, depending on E&M category

■ Example of a Completed PFSH

In the PFSH of the sample patient, all three histories are documented, so the PFSH is complete.

PFSH: The patient has a history of upper respiratory infections but does not report any regular history of throat infections. There are no prior hospitalizations or surgeries. The patient has environmental allergies and no known drug allergies. Immunizations are current. The patient lives with his parents and two siblings, none of whom have been ill with similar symptoms in the recent past. The patient is active in soccer and attends 5th grade regularly.

Past history—upper respiratory infections (medical); no throat infections (medical); no prior hospitalizations or surgeries (surgical); environmental allergies, NKDA (allergies); immunizations current.

Family history—No one in the family has been ill with similar symptoms.

Social history—Lives with his parents and two siblings; active in soccer; 5th grade.

✳ Communicating With Medical Providers

Although the rules for using the ROS shortcut AON are specific, the concept is often misunderstood. Physicians may want to use only a statement such as "all systems negative." This is incorrect because the physician must at least document the problem pertinent system. As well, there is at least one positive system review related to the Chief Complaint, so only stating AON is inaccurate. Another way physicians misuse the shortcut is to insert some number of systems: 8, or 10, or 13, and so on, such as, "A 10 point review of systems was negative." This is a problem because there are 14 systems total. Noting that only 10 were reviewed is fewer than "all" the systems, and the reviewer will not know which 10 of the 14 systems were reviewed. The physician must follow the AON rules exactly in order to use the shortcut. Some practices avoid using it due to the confusion it can cause.

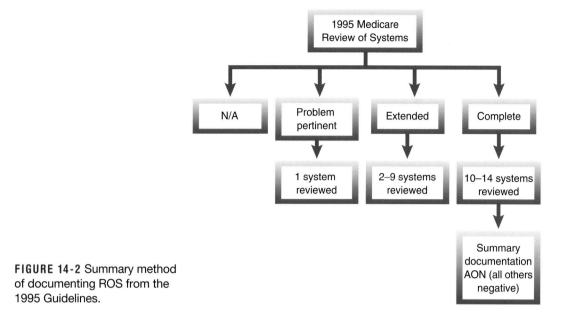

FIGURE 14-2 Summary method of documenting ROS from the 1995 Guidelines.

TABLE 14.3   1995 Guidelines PFSH—Complete by E&M Service Type

2 History Elements Required For:	3 History Elements Required For:
Office or Other Outpatient Services—Established (99911–99215) Emergency Department (99281–99285) Domiciliary...Care Services—Established (99334-99337) Home Services—Established (99347–99350)	Office or Other Outpatient Services—New (99201–99205) Initial Observation Care (99218–99220) Initial Hospital Care (99221–99223) Consultations (99241–99255) Initial Nursing Facility Care (99304–99306) Domiciliary...Care Services—New (99324–99328) Home Services—New (99341–99345)

Finally, the 1995 Guidelines define 4 types of History—Problem Focused, Expanded Problem Focused, Detailed, and Comprehensive. As in CPT, the minimum level of all elements must be met in order to select the appropriate History type. Some elements might exceed the level required, but each one must be met at a minimum. Table 14.4 describes the 4 types of History. Occasionally 2 types of History require the same element level. For example, both Detailed and Comprehensive require an extended HPI. When this occurs, the higher History type, in this case Comprehensive, is credited.

TABLE 14.4   Medicare 1995 Documentation Guidelines History Types and Element Minimums for Each Type*

History Type	Problem Focused	Expanded Problem Focused	Detailed	Comprehensive
Chief Complaint	Required	Required	Required	Required
HPI	Brief (1–3 elements)		Extended (4 or more elements)	
ROS	N/A	Problem Pertinent (1 system)	Extended (2-9 systems)	Complete (10–14 systems)
PFSH	N/A	N/A	Pertinent (1 history)	Complete (2 or 3 histories according to Table 14.3)

*Select the column furthest to left where element minimums are met.

Review the History presented throughout the chapter for the sample patient. There is a Chief Complaint present—Sore throat. HPI is Extended. ROS is Extended. PFSH is Complete. Table 14.5 summarizes the History elements for the sample patient, which is Detailed.

CRITICAL THINKING

If the patient is incapacitated and no family or other representative is available, the physician may document the condition that prevents collecting the History. This counts as History—Comprehensive. Why is a Comprehensive type assumed instead of a Problem Focused type?

■ EXAM

The 1995 Guidelines use the same body areas and organ systems as CPT identifies, as shown on Table 14.6.

Unfortunately, the 1995 Guidelines do not completely resolve the challenge of quantifying the Exam component. There are four types, described in Table 14.7.

Given these definitions, the Exam component remains unclear in a couple of ways. Clearly, a Problem Focused Exam requires examination of one body area or organ system. On the other end of the spectrum, a physician must document an examination of eight or more organ systems for a Comprehensive Exam. However, note that only organ systems may be used to achieve a Comprehensive Exam, not body areas. Documentation of an exam by body area can, at most, result in a Detailed Exam. In between those two

TABLE 14.5   Medicare 1995 Documentation Guidelines History Types and Element Minimums for Each Type*

Example Patient—Detailed History

History Type	Problem Focused	Expanded Problem Focused	Detailed	Comprehensive
Chief Complaint	Required	Required	Required	Required
HPI	Brief (1–3 elements)		**Extended (4 or more elements)**	
ROS	N/A	Problem Pertinent (1 system)	**Extended (2-9 systems)**	Complete (10–14 systems)
PFSH	N/A	N/A	Pertinent (1 history)	**Complete (2 or 3 histories according to Table 14.3)**

*Select the column furthest to left where are element minimums are met.

TABLE 14.6   CPT Body Areas and Organ Systems

CPT Defined Body Areas	CPT Defined Organ Systems
Head, including the face	Eyes
Neck	Ears, nose, mouth, and throat
Chest, including breasts and axillae	Cardiovascular
Abdomen	Respiratory
Genitalia, groin, buttocks	Gastrointestinal
Back	Genitourinary
Each extremity	Musculoskeletal
	Skin
	Neurological
	Psychiatric
	Hematological/lymphatic/immunological

TABLE 14.7 Medicare 1995 Documentation Guidelines Exam Types and Element Minimums for Each Type

Exam Type	Problem Focused	Expanded Problem Focused	Detailed	Comprehensive
	Limited exam of the affected body area or organ system	Limited exam of the affected body area or organ system and other symptomatic or related organ system(s)	Extended exam of the affected body area(s) and other symptomatic or related organ system(s)	General multi-system exam or complete exam of a single organ system

levels are Expanded Problem Focused (EPF) and Detailed Exam, both requiring an examination of 2–7 organ systems. The difference is that EPF includes a "limited" exam and Detailed requires an "extended" exam of the affected body area or organ system.

The guidelines do not provide any additional information on how to identify a limited or extended exam, and payers will set their own definitions of limited and extended, as will many practices. For the purposes of this text, the following definitions will apply:

- An extended exam includes documentation of exam of 2–7 body areas or organ systems with three or more exam details for at least 1 of the documented body areas or organ systems.

- A limited exam includes documentation of exam of 2–7 body areas or organ systems, but no body area or organ system has three or more exam details.

For example, a cardiovascular exam documented as "regular rate and rhythm; no murmurs; no peripheral edema" includes three exam details, making it an extended exam. Documentation of cardiovascular "normal" includes just one exam detail—a limited exam.

Example of a patient exam

Patient is afebrile. No respiratory distress. Pharyngeal exam reveals general erythema, no exudates, minor swelling. Uvula is mid-line. Upon palpation, cervical lymph nodes are enlarged and tender. Gastrointestinal examination reveals no splenomegaly.

General: Patient is afebrile. (Limited)
Head: Atraumatic, normocephalic. Eyes clear. (Limited)
ENMT: Generalized erythema, no exudates, minor swelling. Uvula is mid-line. (Extended)
CV: RRR. (Limited)
Respiratory: Normal. (Limited)
GI: No splenomegaly. (Limited)

To determine the proper level of Exam, first determine how many body area(s) and organ system(s) the physician examined. If the physician examined more than 1 body area or organ system, but fewer than 8 organ systems, the Exam is either EPF or Detailed. At least one of the body areas or organ systems must have three or more Exam details for a Detailed Exam. ENMT (organ system) has three or more Exam details; thus this is a Detailed Exam (See Table 14.8).

MEDICAL DECISION MAKING

Medical Decision Making (MDM) is another area where the 1995 Guidelines allow for interpretation. The 1995 Guidelines define MDM with a qualitative method similar to CPT. In 1994, the 1995 Guidelines were beta-tested at the Marshfield Clinic in Wisconsin. Marshfield Clinic and the

TABLE 14.8 **Medicare 1995 Documentation Guidelines Exam Types and Element Minimums for Each Type**

Example Patient—Detailed

Exam Type	Problem Focused	Expanded Problem Focused	Detailed	Comprehensive
	Limited exam of the affected body area or organ system	Limited exam of the affected body area or organ system and other symptomatic or related organ system(s)	**Extended exam of the affected body area(s) and other symptomatic or related organ system(s)**	General multi-system exam or complete exam of a single organ system (8 or more organ systems)

regional Medicare carrier collaboratively developed a point system for the 1995 Guidelines for MDM in order to quantify the component. Although this point system has never been officially endorsed by Medicare, it is widely used and considered the industry standard.

MDM includes three elements: Number of Diagnoses or Management Options, Amount and/or Complexity of Data to Be Reviewed, and Risk of Complications and/or Morbidity or Mortality. As with CPT, the 1995 Guidelines only require that *any two* of the three element levels be met in order to report the MDM type. A common misconception is that the MDM type cannot be higher than the Risk will allow. However, all three elements have equal weight, and any two of the three can be used to select the MDM type.

Number of Diagnoses and/or Treatment Options

Number of Diagnoses and/or Treatment Options is quantified by assigning points to the type and number of problems addressed during the visit. See Table 14.9 for the enumeration of this element. Only problems addressed during the visit should be counted. For example, if the patient has diabetes but presents with wrist pain, and diabetes is not considered or treated during the visit, then only the wrist pain is credited.

Minor is the lowest level of Diagnoses and/or Treatment Options. Classifying a problem as minor is rather subjective, but it is typically one that needs no intervention by the physician, such as a small, uninfected superficial laceration. If it is not a minor problem, then the coder must determine whether the *problem,* not the patient, is new or established to the treating physician. Do not consider whether the patient has received treatment for the condition elsewhere. For example, the patient may be seeing a specialist for a condition his or her primary care physician could not treat. The problem is new to the specialist. Or a patient may be a long-time patient of a primary care physician but presents for the first time with wrist pain. The problem is new to the primary care physician.

TABLE 14.9 **Medicare 1995 Documentation Guidelines Medical Decision Making**

Number of Diagnoses or Management Options

Diagnoses & Treatment Options	Points per Problem	# of Problems	Maximum Points	Total Points (Points × Problems)
Minor problem	1	× _____	2	
Established problem (to the physician), stable or improving	1	× _____		
Established problem (to the physician), worsening or not improved	2	× _____		
New problem (to the physician), no additional work-up planned	3	× _____	3	
New problem (to the physician), additional work-up planned	4	× _____		
			Total Points =	

For problems established to the physician, the documentation should reflect whether the problem is stable, improving, or worsening. Stable or improving, the second level of Diagnoses and/or Treatment Options, is the default if the documentation is not explicit. For problems new to the physician, the highest levels of Diagnoses and/or Treatment Options, deciding whether additional work-up is planned depends on whether a definitive diagnosis is determined during the visit. To assign points for New Problem, Additional Work-up Planned, the physician is unsure of the diagnosis by the end of the visit and orders additional testing or other care to determine a diagnosis outside of the current visit, as noted in Table 14.9. If the physician determines a definitive diagnosis for a new problem during the visit, no additional information is needed to determine a diagnosis, New Problem No Additional Work-up Planned. The physician might order additional testing during the visit to treat the patient, which is different from ordering additional testing to determine a diagnosis. Ordering treatment is not considered as part of Diagnoses and/or Treatment Options.

Assign the appropriate number of points for every problem treated during the visit. If the patient presents with three conditions, such as headache, fatigue, and cough, assign points for each of the three problems. Note, however, that some point sections have a maximum. No matter how many conditions the patient has that are new diagnoses with no additional work-up planned, only 3 points may be assigned for this category. Total the points from all of the categories to determine the number of diagnoses and/or treatment options.

Example of a documented MDM

The sample patient has the following documented MDM, "Rapid strep positive. Prescribed Amoxicillin t.i.d. 10 days for strep throat. Continue warm salt-water gargle as tolerated. Soft food and ample fluids, slowly reintroduce solid foods. Return to school when fever is resolved and patient is not fatigued."

The patient presented with a sore throat, which is a new problem to the physician. By the end of the visit, the physician determines the patient has strep throat and does not need additional information outside of the visit to determine a diagnosis. This MDM results in one new problem with no additional work-up planned for 3 points (Table 14.10).

Data to Be Reviewed

The second element of MDM is Data to Be Reviewed. The points system for this element considers the additional information and testing the physician considers as part of the decision making process during the visit. Notice that, similar to counting for PFSH, regardless of how many items appear under each section, assign only 1 or 2 points. See Table 14.11 for the enumeration of Data to Be Reviewed.

TABLE 14.10   Medicare 1995 Documentation Guidelines Medical Decision Making

Number of Diagnoses or Management Options
Example Patient

Diagnoses & Treatment Options	Points per Problem	# of Problems	Maximum Points	Total Points (Points × Problems)
Minor problem	1	× _____	2	
Established problem (to the physician), stable or improving	1	× _____		
Established problem (to the physician), worsening or not improved	2	× _____		
New problem (to the physician), no additional work-up planned	**3**	**× 1**	**3**	**3**
New problem (to the physician), additional work-up planned	4	× _____		
			Total Points =	3

TABLE 14.11 Medicare 1995 Documentation Guidelines Medical Decision Making

Data to Be Reviewed

Data	Points per Data Type	Points for This Visit
Laboratory order and/or results review	1	
Radiology order and/or results review	1	
Medicine section of CPT order and/or results review	1	
Discuss test results with the performing physician	1	
Decision to obtain old records and/or history from someone other than the patient	1	
Review and summary of old records and/or obtaining history from someone other than the patient and/or discussion of the case with another provider	2	
Personal review of image, tracing, or specimen (not review of the report)	2	
	Total points =	

Notice that the Laboratory, Radiology, and Medicine items include both ordering and reviewing tests from the CPT sections, regardless of how many tests are considered, and ordering or reviewing those tests result in 1 point. For example, even if the physician orders four laboratory tests, assign just 1 point for Laboratory. The other items in this element must be documented explicitly in order to be assigned a point. For example, to assign points for discussion of the case with another provider, the documentation must note specifically the physician had a phone or face-to-face discussion with the performing provider of a test.

▍ Example of points assigned to test performed in the office

The example patient had a rapid strep test performed in the office. Assign this 1 point for Laboratory ordered and/or reviewed (see Table 14.12).

Risk of Complications and/or Morbidity or Mortality

The third MDM element is Risk of Complications and/or Morbidity or Mortality. The 1995 Guidelines include a Table of Risk that lists examples of the various levels of patient risk. The Table of Risk is shown in Table 14.13 as well as in Appendix A as part of the 1995 Guidelines.

The Table of Risk defines four levels of risk to the patient in three ways—by the nature of the presenting problem, the type of diagnostic procedures ordered, and by the management options selected to treat the

TABLE 14.12 Medicare 1995 Documentation Guidelines Medical Decision Making

Data to Be Reviewed
Example Patient

Data	Points per Data Type	Points for This Visit
Laboratory order and/or results review	**1**	**1**
Radiology order and/or results review	1	
Medicine section of CPT order and/or results review	1	
Discuss test results with the performing physician	1	
Decision to obtain old records and/or history from someone other than the patient	1	
Review and summary of old records and/or obtaining history from someone other than the patient and/or discussion of the case with another provider	2	
Personal review of image, tracing, or specimen (not review of the report)	2	
	Total points =	1

TABLE 14.13 Table of Risk

Level of Risk	Presenting Problem(s)	Diagnostic Procedure(s) Ordered	Management Options Selected
Minimal	• One self-limiting or minor problem, e.g., cold, insect bite, tinea corporis	• Laboratory tests requiring venipuncture • Chest x-rays • EKG/EEG • Urinalysis • Ultrasound, e.g., echocardiography • KOH prep	• Rest • Gargles • Elastic bandages • Superficial dressings
Low	• Two or more self-limiting or minor problems • One stable chronic illness, e.g., well controlled hypertension or non-insulin dependent diabetes, cataract, BPH • Acute uncomplicated illness or injury, eg, cystitis, allergic rhinitis, simple sprain	• Physiologic tests not under stress, e.g., pulmonary function tests • Non-cardiovascular imaging studies with contrast, e.g., barium enema • Superficial needle biopsies • Clinical laboratory tests requiring arterial puncture • Skin biopsies	• Over-the-counter drugs • Minor surgery with no identified risk factors • Physical therapy • Occupational therapy • IV fluids without additives
Moderate	• One or more illnesses with mild exacerbation, progression, or side effects of treatment • Two or more stable chronic illnesses • Undiagnosed new problem with uncertain prognosis, e.g., lump in breast • Acute illness with systemic symptoms, e.g., pyelonephritis, pneumonitis, colitis • Acute complicated injury, e.g., head injury with brief loss of consciousness	• Physiologic tests under stress, e.g., cardiac stress test, fetal contraction stress test • Diagnostic endoscopies with no identified risk factors • Deep needle or incisional biopsy • Cardiovascular imaging studies with contrast and no identified risk factors, e.g., arteriogram, cardiac catheterization • Obtain fluid from body cavity, e.g., lumbar puncture, thoracentesis, culdocentesis	• Minor surgery with identified risk factors • Elective major surgery (open percutaneous or endoscopic) with no identified risk factors • Prescription drug management • Therapeutic nuclear management • IV fluids with additives • Closed treatment of fracture or dislocation without manipulation
High	• One or more chronic illnesses with severe exacerbation, progression, or side effects of treatment • Acute or chronic illnesses or injuries that pose a threat to life or bodily function, e.g., multiple trauma, acute MI, pulmonary embolus, severe respiratory distress, progressive severe rheumatoid arthritis, psychiatric illness with potential threat to self or others, peritonitis, acute renal failure • An abrupt change in neurologic status, e.g., seizure, TIA, weakness, or sensory loss	• Cardiovascular imaging studies with contrast with identified risk factors • Cardiac electrophysiological tests • Diagnostic endoscopies with identified risk factors • Discography	• Elective major surgery (open, percutaneous, or endoscopic) with identified risk factors • Emergency major surgery (open, percutaneous, or endoscopic) • Parenteral controlled substances • Drug therapy requiring intensive monitoring for toxicity • Decision not to resuscitate or to de-escalate care because of poor prognosis

From www.cms.gov/Outreach-and-Education/Medicare-Learning-Network-MLN/MLNEdWebGuide/Downloads/95Docguidelines.pdf.

patient. Note that the items listed are examples, not an exhaustive list. Only one item must be identified from any of the three areas to identify the level of risk. For example, when the patient has an undiagnosed new problem that could have a variety of outcomes, such as a breast lump, assign moderate level risk. The highest risk level with an identified item is the risk associated with the problem being addressed.

> ### ▉ Example of how to use the table of risk
>
> The example patient has strep throat for which an antibiotic is prescribed. Using the Table of Risk, the presenting problem of sore throat is an acute uncomplicated illness, which is low risk. The rapid strep is not an identified diagnostic procedure. The management options selected include prescribing an antibiotic, a moderate risk. The highest item listed presents moderate risk, so the risk for the visit then is moderate.

There are four types of MDM—straightforward, low, moderate, and high. The minimum elements for only two of the three MDM elements must be met to select an MDM level. Review the MDM presented throughout the chapter for the sample patient. There are 3 points for Number of Diagnoses and/or Treatment Options, 1 point for Data to Be Reviewed, and Moderate Risk. Table 14.14 summarizes the MDM elements for the sample patient, which is Moderate.

▉ ASSIGNING AN E&M SUBCATEGORY LEVEL

Having assigned types of History, Exam, and MDM, an E&M level can now be determined. The patient was seen in the physician office and is an established patient. To select an E&M level, the key component minimums must be met for either 2 of 3 or 3 of 3 key components, according to the E&M code description. Office or Other Outpatient Services, Established Patient levels require only 2 of 3 key component minimums. For codes that require only 2 of 3 key component minimums, disregard the lowest component type, and then select the E&M level with the next lowest component type. Put another way, select the E&M level corresponding to the middle component type. In the example in Table 14.15, all 3 element minimums are met for 99214. A reminder that similar to MDM and Risk, a misconception regarding codes that require 2 of 3 key components minimums be met is that the level cannot be higher than the corresponding MDM type. All 3 components have equal weight, and any 2 of the 3 may be used to select the E&M level.

Using an Audit Tool to Assign an E&M Subcategory Level

Many components, elements, and points make up an E&M level. The easiest way to consider all of this information at once is to use an Audit Tool. See Figure 14-3 and Appendix C for a sample audit tool. It is important when using an audit tool to consider all of the components and elements in order. Make multiple copies of the Audit Tool in Appendix C for use in assigning E&M levels in the remainder of this textbook. Practice using the audit tool to assign an E&M level for the sample patient.

TABLE 14.14 Medicare 1995 Documentation Guidelines Medical Decision Making*

Sample Patient—Moderate

	Straightforward	Low	Moderate	High
Number of Diagnoses and/or Treatment Options	1	2	**3**	4+
Data to be Reviewed	**0-1**	2	3	4+
Risk	Minimal	Low	**Moderate**	High

*Select the column second from the left where are element minimums are met.

Professional Charge Audit Worksheet

Patient Name: _____ Provider: _____ DOS: _____

Account Number: _____ Coded: _____ / Audited: _____ Initials: _____

Chief Complaint: _____

History Component				
HPI	1–3		4+	
ROS	0	1	2–9	10+ or 1+AON
PFSH	0	0	1	2/3*
	PF	EPF	D	C

(Choose marked column farthest to the left)

HISTORY

History of Present Illness
○ Location   ○ Quality   ○ Timing   ○ Modifying factors
○ Duration   ○ Severity   ○ Context   ○ Assoc. signs & symptoms

Review of Systems
○ Constitut.   ○ Cardiovasc.   ○ GU   ○ Neuro   ○ Endocrine
○ Eyes   ○ Respiratory   ○ Musculo   ○ Psych   ○ Hem/lymph
○ ENMT   ○ GI   ○ Integument (skin, breast)   ○ Allerg/imm
                         ○ 1 & "All others negative"

Past, Family, Social Histories
○ Past (illnesses, operations, allergies, med list)
○ Family (family medical history as it pertains to the patient's complaints)
○ Social (age-appropriate work, tobacco/alcohol/drugs,
          school and activities, living situation, etc.)

Exam Component				
EXAM	1	2–7L	2–7E	8
	PF	EPF	D	C

PHYSICAL EXAM

Organ Systems
○ Constitut.   ○ Cardiovasc.   ○ GU   ○ Neuro
○ Eyes   ○ Respiratory   ○ Musculo   ○ Psych
○ ENMT   ○ GI   ○ Integument   ○ Hem/lymph/imm

Body Areas - *generally use only for major trauma*
○ Head   ○ Chest   ○ Genital/area   ○ Left arm   ○ Left leg
○ Neck   ○ Abdomen   ○ Back/spine   ○ Right arm   ○ Right leg
                              ○ Unspecified extremity(s)

Decision Making Component				
Diag	1	2	3	4+
Data	0–1	2	3	4+
Risk	Min	Low	Mod	High
	SF	Low	Mod	High

(Choose middle marked column)

MEDICAL DECISION MAKING

Diagnosis & Treatment Options (problem is new/est to the provider)
1 Minor problem   X _____ = max 2
1 Established problem, stable or improving   X _____ = _____
2 Established problem, worsening or not improv.   X _____ = _____
3 New problem, no additional work-up planned   X _____ = max 3*
4 New problem, additional work-up planned   X _____ = _____

Data to be Reviewed   (listed points, regardless of number of tests)
1 Lab order *and/or* review
1 Radiology order *and/or* review
1 Medicine section of CPT *order and/or* review
1 Discuss test results with performing physician
1 Decision to obtain old records *and/or* history from someone other than patient
2 Review & summary of old records *and/or* obtain hx from non-patient
   and/or discussion of case with another provider
2 Personal review of image, tracing, or specimen - not review of report

○ Minimal   ○ Low   ○ Moderate   ○ High
(See Table of Risk)

OP New/Consults					
Hist.	PF	EPF	D	C	C
Exam	PF	EPF	D	C	C
MDM	SF	SF	L	M	H
	1	2	3	4	5

(Choose marked column farthest to the left)

OP Established					
Hist.		PF	EPF	D	C
Exam		PF	EPF	D	C
MDM		SF	L	M	H
	1	2	3	4	5

(Choose middle marked column)

Emergency Department					
Hist.	PF	EPF	EPF	D	C
Exam	PF	EPF	EPF	D	C
MDM	SF	L	M	M	H
	1	2	3	4	5

(Choose marked column farthest to the left)

Initial Hospital/Obsrv			
Hist.	D	C	C
Exam	D	C	C
MDM	L	M	H
	1	2	3

(Choose marked column to the left)

Sub Hospital/Obsrv			
Hist.	PF	EPF	D
Exam	PF	EPF	D
MDM	L	M	H
	1	2	3

(Choose middle marked column)

*Complete PFSH: 3 - New OP, Consults, Initial hosp care, hosp observ; 2 - Est OP, Emergency; None - Sub Hosp/Obsrv/NF

FIGURE 14-3 Audit Tool.

TABLE 14.15 Summary of Sample Patient Visit Documentation

E/M Subcategory Level	History	Exam	Medical Decision Making	Meet Requirements? (At least two of the three key component minimums are met.)
99211	Does not require the presence of a physician.			Yes
99212	Problem focused	Problem focused	Straightforward	Yes
99213	Expanded problem focused	Expanded problem focused	Low	Yes
99214	**Detailed**	**Detailed**	**Moderate**	Yes
99215	Comprehensive	Comprehensive	High	No

Remember to complete all of the steps in assigning an E&M subcategory level. Skipping any element can lead to assigning the wrong code.

1. Identify the E&M Category

2. Determine whether the patient is new or established and if that will affect the E&M subcategory.

3. Identify the correct History type:
   a. Identify the Chief Complaint.
   b. Identify the HPI.
   c. Identify the ROS.
   d. Identify the PFSH.

4. Identify the correct Exam type.

5. Identify the correct MDM type:
   a. Identify the Number of Diagnoses and/or Management Options.
   b. Identify the Data to Be Reviewed.
   c. Identify the level of Risk.

6. Consider whether the E&M subcategory requires 2 or 3 element minimums be met.

7. Assign the E&M level.

●●● SUMMARY

- In the 1995 Guidelines, HPI—Brief includes 1–3 elements and HPI—Extended includes 4 or more elements.
- Four types of ROS are defined—N/A, Problem Pertinent (1 system), Extended (2–9 systems), Complete (10–14 systems).
- When all 14 systems are reviewed, the problem pertinent system, any *problem pertinent* negatives, and all positive systems must be documented. The remaining systems may be abbreviated "all others negative (AON)".
- The 1995 Guidelines include four types of Exam—Problem focused (1 organ system or body area), Expanded problem focused (2–7 organ systems or body areas), Detailed (2–7 organ systems or body areas), and Comprehensive (8 or more organ systems).
- For text exercises, a Detailed Exam includes at least 1 body area or organ system with at least three details listed for that body area or organ system.
- In MDM, Number of Diagnoses and/or Treatment Options is quantified by how many problems the physician treats and whether the problems are new to the physician.
- Data to Be Reviewed is enumerated by the types of data ordered and/or reviewed.
- The Table of Risk determines the patient's risk of complications and/or morbidity or mortality.
- An audit tool condenses the information necessary to assign an E&M level into an efficient method for coding.

Chapter Review Exercises

1. Assign the correct History type for a note including 4 HPI elements, 10 systems of review, and 3 PFSH. The patient is new and seen in the physician office.

2. Assign the correct History type for a note including 4 HPI elements, 5 systems of review, and 1 PFSH. The patient is new and seen in the physician office.

3. Assign the correct Exam type for a note including the following organ systems—constitutional, eye, ENMT, cardiovascular, respiratory, musculoskeletal, integumentary, and GI.

4. Assign the correct Exam type for a note including the following body areas and organ systems: Head—normocephalic, atraumatic, no steps; Neck—trachea midline, tissues soft, no lymphadenopathy, no skin changes; Cardiovascular—RRR, no rubs, no murmurs.

5. Assign the correct MDM type for the following visit: a new problem to the physician with additional work-up, reviewed lab and ordered radiology, and an undiagnosed problem with uncertain prognosis.

6. Assign the correct MDM type for the following visit: an established problem to the physician that is worsening and an established problem to the physician that is stable, reviewed radiology and medicine tests and ordered laboratory, and the patient has a chronic illness with mild exacerbation, laboratory tests requiring venipuncture, and elective major surgery with identified risk factors was scheduled.

7. Using an audit tool, complete the steps to assign an E&M subcategory level. The visit information follows the steps to be answered.
   a. Identify the E&M Category.
   b. Determine whether the patient is new or established and if that will affect the E&M subcategory.
   c. Identify the correct History type:
      i. Identify if a Chief Complaint is documented.
      ii. Identify the HPI.
      iii. Identify the ROS.
      iv. Identify the PFSH.
   d. Identify the correct Exam type.
   e. Identify the correct MDM type:
      i. Identify the Number of Diagnoses and/or Management Options.
      ii. Identify the Data to Be Reviewed.
      iii. Identify the level of Risk.
   f. Consider whether the E&M subcategory requires 2 or 3 element minimums be met.
   g. Assign the E&M level.

   Use this information to answer each step:
      i. The patient was seen in the physician office.
      ii. The patient has not been seen by the practice in the last 3 years.
      iii. The physician documents a Chief Complaint and HPI including location and duration.
      iv. 8 systems are reviewed.
      v. PSFH is noted.
      vi. The physical exam is brief, including one detail for ENMT and one detail for Eye.

177

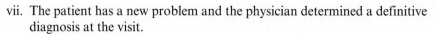

vii. The patient has a new problem and the physician determined a definitive diagnosis at the visit.

viii. The physician ordered lab tests and x-rays and decided to order the patient's old records from another practice.

ix. The patient has a stable chronic illness.

x. The tests the physician ordered include an incisional biopsy.

xi. The physician chose only to treat the problem for today with OTC drugs.

8. Using an audit tool, complete the steps to assign an E&M subcategory level. The visit information follows the steps to be answered:

a. Identify the E&M Category.

b. Determine whether the patient is new or established and if that will affect the E&M subcategory.

c. Identify the correct History type:

i. Identify if a Chief Complaint is documented.

ii. Identify the HPI.

iii. Identify the ROS.

iv. Identify the PFSH.

d. Identify the correct Exam type.

e. Identify the correct MDM type:

i. Identify the Number of Diagnoses and/or Management Options.

ii. Identify the Data to Be Reviewed.

iii. Identify the level of Risk.

f. Consider whether the E&M subcategory requires 2 or 3 element minimums be met.

g. Assign the E&M level.

Use this information to answer each step:

i. The patient was seen in the hospital on the first day of an inpatient stay.

ii. The patient was last seen a week ago in the office.

iii. The physician documents a Chief Complaint and HPI including location, duration, context, and modifying factors.

iv. 10 systems are reviewed.

v. PFSH is noted.

vi. The physical exam includes the following organ systems: constitutional, eye, ENMT, cardiovascular, respiratory, musculoskeletal, integumentary, neurological, psychological, and hematological.

vii. The patient has 3 established problems—2 worsening and 1 stable.

viii. The physician ordered lab and x-ray, talked to physician who performed a diagnostic heart cath, and talked to a cardiac surgeon about whether the patient was a surgical candidate.

ix. The patient has one or more chronic illnesses with mild exacerbation.

x. The tests the physician ordered include cardiovascular imaging studies with contrast and no identified risk factors

xi. The physician chose to treat the problem with elective major surgery with no identified risk factors.

9. Using an audit tool, complete the steps to assign an E&M subcategory level. The visit information follows the steps to be answered:

   a. Identify the E&M Category.

   b. Determine whether the patient is new or established and if that will affect the E&M subcategory.

   c. Identify the correct History type.

      i. Identify if a Chief Complaint is documented.

      ii. Identify the HPI.

      iii. Identify the ROS.

      iv. Identify the PFSH.

   d. Identify the correct Exam type.

   e. Identify the correct MDM type:

      i. Identify the Number of Diagnoses and/or Management Options.

      ii. Identify the Data to Be Reviewed.

      iii. Identify the level of Risk.

   f. Consider whether the E&M subcategory requires 2 or 3 element minimums be met.

   g. Assign the E&M level.

   Use this information to answer each step:

      i. The patient was seen in the physician office.

      ii. The patient was last seen in the office about a year ago.

      iii. The physician documents a Chief Complaint and HPI including location.

      iv. 1 problem pertinent system is reviewed.

      v. Past history is documented.

      vi. The physical exam includes the following organ systems: constitutional, eye, ENMT, cardiovascular, respiratory, musculoskeletal, integumentary, neurological, psychological, and hematological.

      vii. The patient has a new problem, and the physician needs to order additional tests to determine a diagnosis.

      viii. The physician ordered lab, x-ray, and medicine tests.

      ix. The patient has an undiagnosed new problem with an uncertain prognosis.

      x. The tests the physician ordered include chest x-rays.

      xi. As there is no diagnosis yet, the physician did not select any management options.

10. Using an audit tool, complete the steps to assign an E&M subcategory level. The visit information follows the steps to be answered:

    a. Identify the E&M Category.

    b. Determine whether the patient is new or established and if that will affect the E&M subcategory.

    c. Identify the correct History type:

       i. Identify if a Chief Complaint is documented

       ii. Identify the HPI.

       iii. Identify the ROS.

       iv. Identify the PFSH.

    d. Identify the correct Exam type.

    e. Identify the correct MDM type.

   i. Identify the Number of Diagnoses and/or Management Options.
   ii. Identify the Data to Be Reviewed.
   iii. Identify the level of Risk.
f. Consider whether the E&M subcategory requires 2 or 3 element minimums be met.
g. Assign the E&M level.

Use this information to answer each step:

   i. The patient was seen in the Emergency Department.
   ii. The patient has never been seen in this Emergency Department before.
   iii. The physician documents a Chief Complaint and HPI including location, duration, context, and severity.
   iv. All systems are reviewed and properly documented.
   v. Past history is documented.
   vi. The physical exam includes the following body areas: head, neck, chest, back, abdomen, genitalia, all four extremities. The head and neck both include three details of exam.
   vii. The patient has multiple problems new to the physician. The physician determines diagnoses for them and refers the patient to a specialist for admission.
   viii. The physician ordered and reviewed multiple laboratory tests and x-rays.
   ix. The physician personally reviewed the chest x-rays.
   x. The patient has an acute injury that poses a threat to life or bodily function.
   xi. The physician started the patient on IV fluids with additives before turning the patient over to the specialist.

CASE STUDY

Using an audit tool, complete the steps to assign an E&M subcategory level.

[This is the first time Mr. Kim has seen Dr. Bellkey. He is seen in her office in a downtown medical building.]

Mr. Kim is a 35-year-old welder by trade who was found to have borderline glucose levels during a hospital stay 1 month ago. The levels were higher after meals but never exceeded 200 mg/dL. The patient thinks he might have experienced some frequent urination, but that could be from increased fluid intake. Since his hospital stay, the patient has been concerned about his blood sugar and has started walking 20 minutes at least 5 days/week and reducing his caloric intake.

Mr. Kim reports no recent weight changes or changes in appetite. His vision has returned to normal since his corneal transplant. He hasn't noticed any recent cuts or bruises that are slow to heal. No extremity tingling or numbness. No oral infections. No skin infections. No bladder infections. Normal bowel movements. No shortness of breath, no chest pains. Patient reports his knees hurt from time to time from remote history of athletics, but the pain is controlled with ibuprofen. No depression, slight anxiety concerning healing eye trauma. No other current endocrine symptoms or disease. Patient is immunosuppressed due to the corneal transplant and reports his medication is preventing rejection.

Patient has recent surgical history of corneal transplant without complication. Is immunosuppressed. No other medications. Patient reports paternal grandfather developed type II diabetes over 60. No other diabetic history. Patient is a welder and has recently started an exercise routine.

Exam:
Head: normocephalic, atraumatic
Neck: supple, trachea midline, no lymphadenopathy
Eyes: grossly normal
ENMT: mucous membranes pink
Cardiovascular: RRR
Respiratory: clear breath sounds bilateral
GI: Postive bowel sounds, no organomegaly
GU: external genitalia normal, no hernias palpated
Extremities: full ROM in all four extremities; positive reflexes and strength × 4; no skin changes noted
Neuro: cranial nerves II–XII normal; patient is oriented × 3
Data Reviewed:
Patient had a fasting blood sugar three days ago 90 mg/dL, which is high normal.
Cholesterol also elevated, but WNL.
Other labs were normal.
Assessment and Plan:
Mr. Kim had recent elevated blood sugars, but latest test shows high normal. At this time I would not consider him diabetic or pre-diabetic, given his absence of symptoms and transient blood sugar levels. Mr. Kim should continue his new diet and exercise habits. I gave him a pamphlet today on healthy eating. Mr. Kim should see me every six months to monitor his progress and hopefully avoid any disease process. Should his blood sugars start to increase, we will revisit his diagnosis and treatment. At this

Continued

CASE STUDY—cont'd

point, I think Mr. Kim has a moderate risk of developing type II diabetes at some point in the future.

1. Identify the E&M Category.

2. Determine whether the patient is new or established, and if that will affect the E&M subcategory.

3. Identify the correct History type:
   a. Identify if a Chief Complaint is documented
   b. Identify the HPI.
   c. Identify the ROS.
   d. Identify the PFSH.

4. Identify the correct Exam type.

5. Identify the correct MDM type:
   a. Identify the Number of Diagnoses and/or Management Options.
   b. Identify the Data to Be Reviewed.
   c. Identify the level of Risk.

6. Consider whether the E&M subcategory requires 2 or 3 element minimums be met.

7. Assign the E&M level.

15

Medicare 1997 Documentation Guidelines

Chapter Outline

I. Rationale for the Medicare 1997 Documentation Guidelines
   A. 1997 Guidelines History
   B. 1997 Guidelines Exam
II. 1997 Guidelines Medical Decision Making and Other Components
III. Selecting 1995 Guidelines or 1997 Guidelines

LEARNING OUTCOMES

On completion of this chapter, you will be able to:

1. Assign an Evaluation and Management (E&M) service level using the Medicare 1997 Documentation Guidelines.
2. Distinguish the differences between CPT, Medicare 1995 Documentation Guidelines, and Medicare 1997 Documentation Guidelines.
3. Use an audit tool to assign an E&M service level.

It soon became apparent that the Exam level requirements in the Medicare 1995 Documentation Guidelines (1995 Guidelines) were inadequate for many specialties. Medicare developed another set of guidelines in 1997 (1997 Guidelines) and made two changes: History of Present Illness (HPI) and Exam. This chapter describes the differences between the 1995 and 1997 Guidelines, how to assign an E&M service level based on the 1997 Guidelines, and how to determine which set of guidelines to use.

Focus Questions

How do the 1997 Exam level requirements differ from the 1995 Exam level requirements?

Physicians in which specialties benefit from using the 1997 Guidelines instead of the 1995 Guidelines?

When may a physician choose to use the 1995 or 1997 Guidelines?

RATIONALE FOR THE MEDICARE 1997 DOCUMENTATION GUIDELINES

When Medicare published the 1995 Guidelines, it quickly became evident that, with the many questions surrounding how to use the Exam component of the guidelines, the process remained too subjective for practices to apply them consistently. As well, the general nature of the Exam was not adequate for specialty physicians. An otolaryngologist might perform a complete examination of the patient's head, which would then count as one body area examined. This limited Exam element prevented specialty physicians from reporting appropriate high-level services. Medicare soon decided to make another attempt at E&M guidelines.

1997 Guidelines History

A concept added to the 1997 Guidelines considered care for chronic illness. In lieu of four or more elements of HPI, the physician may achieve an extended HPI by noting the current status of three or more chronic or inactive illnesses. This concept does not apply to a brief HPI. The coder should not apply this concept when using the 1995 Guidelines, as elements of the two sets of guidelines should not be mixed. The History component of the 1997 Guidelines is otherwise unchanged from the 1995 Guidelines.

 CRITICAL THINKING

Why does the status of three chronic illnesses result in an extended HPI?

1997 Guidelines Exam

The 1997 Guidelines Exam is a significantly more exacting Exam component than the 1995 Guidelines Exam. The requirements for each Exam type are quite clear. However, the requirements can sometimes seem too exacting for many providers. There are eleven different examination guidelines from which to choose—ten Single-System Exams and a General Multi-System Exam. Any physician may use any of the Exam guidelines.

The Single-System examination guidelines are:

Cardiovascular

Ear, Nose, and Throat

Eye

Genitourinary

Hematological/Lymphatic/Immunological

Musculoskeletal

Neurological

Psychiatric

Respiratory

Skin

Review the 11 Exam guidelines in the 1997 Guidelines in Appendix B. Notice the layout and configuration of each Exam, how they differ, and how they are similar. Each Exam includes multiple body areas and organ systems with bullet point Exam elements. Some of those body areas or organ systems are shaded, and different body areas or organ systems are shaded from Exam to Exam. The requirements for each exam type are listed on the last page of the particular examination guidelines.

Similar to the 1995 Guidelines, there are four types of Exam in the 1997 Guidelines—Problem Focused, Expanded Problem Focused, Detailed, and Comprehensive. The Exam type requirements vary for each system examination. In general, count the Exam elements by bullet point as listed in the examination guidelines as well as whether the bullet point is from a shaded or unshaded box. The points required for each Exam type are detailed in Table 15.1.

Unless otherwise specified, the physician must document the entire bullet point to count toward the Exam. Complete understanding of the bullet point requirements is necessary to accurately count a

TABLE 15.1   Required Exam Type Elements by Exam

Exam Type	General Multi-System	Single-System	Psychiatric & Eye
Problem Focused	One bullet point from one body area or organ system	One bullet point from one body area or organ system	One bullet point from one body area or organ system
Expanded Problem Focused	Six bullet points from one or more body areas or organ systems	Six bullet points from one or more body areas or organ systems	Six bullet points from one or more body areas or organ systems
Detailed	Two bullet points from each of six systems or twelve bullet points in two *or* more body areas or organ systems	Twelve bullet points from one or more body areas or organ systems	Nine bullet points from one or more body areas or organ systems
Comprehensive	All bullet points in each of at least nine body areas or organ systems *and* at least two bullet points from each of nine body areas or organ systems	All bullet points from all shaded body areas or organ systems *and* at least one bullet point from every unshaded body area or organ system	All bullet points from all shaded body areas or organ systems *and* at least one bullet point from every unshaded body area or organ system

1997 Exam. The following explanations on how to properly use the 1997 Guidelines are also listed in the 1997 Guidelines. Reference the 1997 Guidelines frequently while reading the text.

In the Constitutional element, the bullet point requires documentation of at least three of the seven listed measurements in order to count the bullet point. The bullet point is counted only once, not once for every measurement. If only two measurements are documented, do not give credit for the bullet point. If all seven are documented, credit one bullet point.

When a bullet point includes the terms "and," "and/or," or "any," the physician needs only to document one of the listed terms to count the bullet point. For example, in the General Multi-System Exam, under Eye, the first bullet point, "Inspection of conjunctivae and lids," requires inspection only of the conjunctivae *or* the lids to credit the bullet point. If both conjunctivae *and* lids are examined, credit one bullet point.

Parenthetical examples, often beginning "e.g.," are meant to be examples only. All items listed in the parenthetical examples do not need to be documented. As well, the physician may document an unlisted item that satisfies the bullet point. For example, in the General Multi-System Exam, under Ear, Nose, Mouth, and Throat, the third bullet point is "Assessment of hearing (e.g., whispered voice, finger rub, tuning fork)." The physician may satisfy the bullet point by documenting any hearing assessment method, not just those listed as examples. The physician may also simply document, "hearing normal" to satisfy the bullet. Regardless of the number of methods used to assess hearing, only credit one bullet point.

If the bullet point includes the term "when indicated," the bullet point is required only when there is medical necessity for the Exam element. For example, in the General Multi-System Exam, under Gastrointestinal (Abdomen), the fourth bullet point is, "Examination (when indicated) of anus, perineum and rectum, including sphincter tone, presence of hemorrhoids, rectal masses." The physician does not need to document that the element was not indicated. It is left to the physician's professional discretion whether to examine the body area. If the bullet point is not indicated, and therefore not documented, ignore it when developing any Exam type. Likewise, the physician does not need to document the indications. Documenting the examination itself is sufficient.

In the General Multi-System Exam, under Lymph, there is the notation, "Palpation of lymph nodes in two or more areas:" and a list of areas follows. If the physician documents palpation of only one area, then the non-Comprehensive Exam type receives one bullet point credit. For the Comprehensive Exam type, palpation of any two of the listed areas satisfies the requirement for all elements under Lymph.

In the Musculoskeletal Single-System Exam, there are two special notations. The first is under the Musculoskeletal organ system element. For a Comprehensive Exam type, the physician must document all four bullet points in at least four of the six listed body areas. For the other Exam types, count every bullet point individually. For example, documentation of all four bullet points for the right upper extremity counts as four bullet points. As well, documentation of range of motion assessment in all four extremities counts as four bullet points. The second special note in the Musculoskeletal Single-System Exam is under Skin. For a Comprehensive Exam type, the physician must document skin examination in four of the six listed body areas. For the other Exam types, count every body area individually.

▇ Example patient exam

Patient is afebrile. No respiratory distress. Pharyngeal exam reveals general erythema, no exudates, minor swelling. Uvula is mid-line. Upon palpation, cervical lymph nodes are enlarged and tender. Gastrointestinal examination reveals no splenomegaly.

Try using the General Multi-System Exam, the Respiratory Single-System Exam, and the Ear, Nose, and Throat Single-System Exam to develop the Exam type under the 1997 Guidelines for this patient.

Using the Ear, Nose, and Throat Single-System Exam, determine how many bullet points are satisfied, whether those bullet points are in shaded boxes, and whether it is possible to complete a Comprehensive Exam type.

There is not a Constitutional bullet point, because at least three of the seven vital signs must be measured. Only temperature, "Patient is afebrile," is documented.

Respiratory—Count one bullet point, Inspection of chest, for, "No respiratory distress," which is assessment of respiratory effort.

Ears, Nose, Mouth, and Throat—Count one bullet point for examination of oropharynx: "Pharyngeal exam reveals general erythema, no exudates, minor swelling. Uvula is mid-line."

Lymph—Count one bullet point for palpation of lymph nodes: "Upon palpation, cervical lymph nodes are enlarged and tender."

There are no Gastrointestinal bullet points available under this Single-System exam to account for "no splenomegaly."

Following the instructions for this Exam, there are three documented bullet points, resulting in a Problem Focused Exam.

 CRITICAL THINKING

Do any of the other system exams result in a higher Exam for the 1997 Guidelines?

▇ 1997 GUIDELINES MEDICAL DECISION MAKING AND OTHER COMPONENTS

Medical Decision Making (MDM) is unchanged from the 1995 Guidelines. Time-based documentation and the contributing components are also unchanged.

▇ SELECTING 1995 GUIDELINES OR 1997 GUIDELINES

When Medicare published the 1997 Guidelines, general physicians found the Exam requirements overly strict. Due to lack of consensus on either set of guidelines, Medicare eventually announced that a physician could use either set of guidelines. The physician may select the guidelines that are most advantageous in selecting an E&M level. The physician may also vary the set of guidelines used from visit to visit, although common practice is to select one set of guidelines and use them consistently. The guidelines may not be mixed for the same visit; chronic conditions may not satisfy the HPI when using 1995 Guidelines for Exam. It is important to read the 1997 Guidelines in their entirety (see Appendix B) as well as to compare the two sets of guidelines.

Comparing exam types and the resulting E&M level

The sample patient History is Detailed, and MDM is Moderate under both sets of guidelines.

Using the 1995 Guidelines, the Exam type was Detailed, resulting in a 99214.

Using the 1997 Guidelines, the Exam type was Problem Focused. Because an Office or Other Outpatient Services, Established visit does not require all three component minimums to be met, the visit is still a 99214.

However, if this were a New patient visit, in which all three component minimums must be met, see Table 15.2 for a comparison of the resulting levels. Using the 1995 Guidelines is clearly advantageous, resulting in an E&M level two levels higher than using 1997 Guidelines.

TABLE 15.2   Comparison of 1995 Guidelines and 1997 Guidelines E/M Level

1995 Guidelines—99203

	99201	99202	99203	99204	99204
History	Problem Focused	Expanded Problem Focused	**Detailed**	Comprehensive	Comprehensive
Exam	Problem Focused	Expanded Problem Focused	**Detailed**	Comprehensive	Comprehensive
MDM	Straight-forward	Straight-forward	Low	**Moderate**	High

1997 Guidelines—99201

	99201	99202	99203	99204	99205
History	Problem Focused	Expanded Problem Focused	**Detailed**	Comprehensive	Comprehensive
Exam	**Problem Focused**	Expanded Problem Focused	Detailed	Comprehensive	Comprehensive
MDM	Straight-forward	Straight-forward	Low	**Moderate**	High

The coder may develop the Exam type under both sets of guidelines and determine the highest E&M level that may be assigned.

Typically, coders find that only specialists benefit from using the 1997 Guidelines. Most primary care physicians and many secondary care physicians use the 1995 Guidelines. However, as noted previously, the physician may use either set of guidelines at any time. The novice coder benefits from developing the Exam type using both sets of guidelines.

✳ Communicating With Medical Providers

Some specialists become convinced that they should, or even must, use the 1997 Guidelines for the most benefit to their practice. However, the 1995 Guidelines are often more beneficial. It is valuable to review with the physician typical examinations for the practice using both sets of guidelines and determine which is best for the practice. Physician documentation and needs vary widely from practice to practice and even physician to physician. Both sets of guidelines should be considered for every practice, and occasionally reviewed to consider whether the practice is using the best set.

●●○ S U M M A R Y

- The 1997 Guidelines were created as a result of complaints that the 1995 Guidelines Exam was too vague and favored general physicians.
- The 1997 Guidelines Extended HPI may also be the current status of three chronic or inactive conditions.
- Eleven Exams—General Multi-System and ten Single-System exams.
- Counted by bullet point and shaded boxes.
- Understand the requirements of each bullet point.
- MDM unchanged from 1995 Guidelines.
- Any physician may use any of the Exams.
- The physician may select the guidelines that result in the most advantageous E&M level.
- Without mixing the guidelines within a single visit, the physician may use either set of guidelines for any visit.
- Common practice is to select the guidelines that are most commonly advantageous and to apply them consistently within the practice.

Chapter Review Exercises

1. Assign the correct Exam type using the Respiratory Single-System Exam for a note including twelve bullet points.

2. Assign the correct Exam type using the Psychiatric Single-System Exam for a note including nine bullet points.

3. Assign the correct Exam type using the General Multi-System Exam for a note including twelve bullet points all in the musculoskeletal system.

4. How many bullet points are assigned using the Hematological/Lymphatic/Immunological Single-System Exam for a note including three vital signs, general appearance of the patient, palpation of the face, examination of the neck, examination of the liver and spleen, palpation of the inguinal lymph nodes, and inspection of the skin?

5. How many bullet points are assigned using the Eye Single-System Exam for a note including gross visual fields, examination of the pupils and irises, measurement of intraocular pressures, documentation of three vital signs, and orientation to person, place, and time?

6. How many bullet points are assigned using the Psychiatric Single-System Exam for a note including three vital signs, examination of gait and station, logical thought process, no suicidal ideation, good insight, oriented ×3, slightly depressed.

7. Develop an Exam type using the Skin Single-System Examination for this note excerpt: "Wt 175. BP 125/76. Pulse 69. Afebrile. Conjunctivae clear. Lips, teeth, and gums appear normal. No evidence of infection in the pharynx. No edema. Hair patterns on head and torso normal. No rashes, lesions, or ulcers noted on the patient's head, neck, chest, abdomen, back, or left upper extremity. Right upper extremity shows diffuse rash. Patient is oriented ×3."

8. Develop an Exam type using the Cardiovascular Single-System Exam for this note excerpt: "Sitting b/p 143/92. Supine blood pressure unchanged. Pulse 85. Temp 97.8. Wt 103. Patient is thin and in no apparent distress. Jugular veins normal. No thyroid enlargement. No respiratory effort. Breath sounds normal bilateral. RRR. Bruit detected in right carotid. Pedal pulses normal. No edema. No cyanosis noted in nails."

9. Using the Genitourinary Single-System Exam for a male patient, note a set of bullet points that would satisfy the requirements for a Comprehensive Exam type. Note each required bullet. Where there is an option, select a bullet. (List just the main point of the bullet.)

10. Using the Neurological Single-System Exam, note a set of bullet points that would satisfy the requirements for a Comprehensive Exam type. Note each required bullet. Where there is an option, select a bullet. (List just the main point of the bullet.)

CASE STUDY

1. Consider the best 1997 Guidelines Exam to use to develop an Exam type for the following patient. Consider trying more than one Exam, and compare the results.

2. Total the noted bullet points.

3. Total the areas/systems with at least one bullet point noted.

4. Total the areas/systems with at least two bullet points noted.

5. Develop the Exam type.

6. Compare the Exam type to the Exam type developed in Chapter 14 using the 1995 Guidelines Exam, and determine which guidelines are most advantageous to use for this visit.

[This is the first time Mr. Kim has seen Dr. Bellkey. He goes to see her in her office in a downtown medical building.]

Mr. Kim is a 35-year-old welder by trade who was found to have borderline glucose levels during a hospital stay 1 month ago.
Exam:
Head: normocephalic, atraumatic
Neck: supple, trachea midline, no lymphadenopathy
Eyes: grossly normal
ENMT: mucous membranes pink
Cardiovascular: RRR
Respiratory: clear breath sounds bilateral
GI: positive bowel sounds, no organomegaly
GU: external genitalia normal, no hernias palpated
Extremities: full ROM in all four extremities; positive reflexes and strength ×4; no skin changes noted
Neuro: cranial nerves II–XII normal; patient is oriented ×3

Case Studies

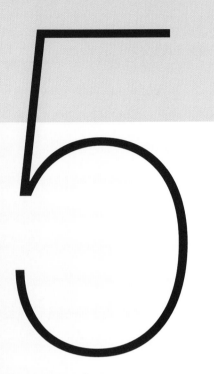

On completion of this unit, you will be able to:

1. Follow the steps to abstract an E&M service code from documentation.
2. Use an audit tool effectively.
     The best way to learn how to code Evaluation and Management (E&M) services is through practice. Using all of the information in this textbook, the Case Study section gives the
student coder the opportunity to practice coding E&M services on real world notes. The practice notes are divided into three sections: Basic, Intermediate, and Advanced.

Directions

Make multiple copies of the Audit Tool on the next page. Use those copies to help you assign accurate E&M levels to the case studies in Unit 5 and any other time you need to assign an E&M level.

A copy of the Audit Tool and also the E&M Subcategory Questionnaire are available online at http://davisplus.fadavis.com, keyword, Brame.

Using an audit tool, complete the steps to assign an E&M subcategory level. The visit information follows the steps to be answered. Your instructors can find answers for all seven steps for coding these case studies in the Instructor's Guide.

Subcategory Questions

1. Identify the E&M Category
2. Determine whether the patient is new or established, and if that will affect the E&M subcategory.
3. Identify the correct History type
   a) Identify the Chief Complaint
   b) Identify the HPI
   c) Identify the ROS
   d) Identify the PFSH
4. Identify the correct Exam type
5. Identify the correct MDM type
   a) Identify the Number of Diagnoses and/or Management Options
   b) Identify the Data to be Reviewed
   c) Identify the level of Risk
6. Consider whether the E&M subcategory requires two or three element minimums be met.
7. Assign the E&M level

E&M Subcategory Questionnaire
Use a copy of this sheet to help you assign an E&M level for each case in this unit.

1. E&M Category _____

2. Patient Type and Effect on E&M Subcategory

   ■ Patient Type   ☐ New   ☐ Established

   ■ Has an effect on E&M subcategory   ☐ Yes   ☐ No

3. History type _____

   ■ CC _____

   ■ HPI _____

   ■ ROS _____

   ■ PFSH _____

4. Exam Type _____

5. MDM Type _____

   ■ Number of Diagnosis and Management Options _____

   ■ Data to be Reviewed _____

   ■ Risk Level _____

6. Number of element minimums _____

7. E&M Level _____

■ BASIC

Note 1

CC: Comedopapular acne

HPI
James is a 15-year-old male who presents with his mother to my office for the first time today for evaluation of chronic comedopapular acne. The acne is diffuse across the patient's face, chest, and back. The condition started with the onset of puberty at approximately age 12. The patient has tried many over the counter medications without adequate result. The acne is often itchy.

ROS
Skin: itching with acne

Constitutional: no recent weight loss

Respiratory: no problems breathing

Musculoskeletal: no joint pain or achiness

History
Patient reports no known drug allergies.

Exam
Constitutional: the patient appears pleasant and in no acute distress

Eyes: clear

ENMT: mucous membranes pink and moist

Neck: supple, no lymphadenopathy

Skin: facial skin shows a diffuse profusion of comedopapular acne, which extends down the neck, across the chest to approximately the nipple line, and down the thoracic back. Some areas show early scarring, especially where the patient notes repeated disturbance of lesions by scratching and expression. The acne does not extend down the arms or otherwise on the body. On the upper back, larger lesions are painful when the surrounding skin is palpated.

Diagnosis
15-year-old pubescent male with diffuse comedopapular acne.

Data reviewed
None

Treatment plan
Due the extent of the patient's acne and its resistance to other remedies, I recommend the patient begin an Accutane regimen. The risks and benefits of this medication were reviewed with the patient and his mother. They were agreeable and eager to begin the treatment plan. Prescription was transmitted to the patient's pharmacy. I will see James back in the office in 8 weeks.

Note 2

CC: Rheumatoid arthritis

HPI

Mary is a 72-year-old new patient who presents to the office today with a long history of rheumatoid arthritis, diagnosed at age 11. Pain is worst in her hands and feet. She currently takes only over the counter pain relievers. She has previously been on a variety of infusion drugs, which were moderately beneficial, but she is no longer able to tolerate these or other RA targeted treatments. She reports some AM stiffness.

ROS

Constitutional: sleeping well

Cardiovascular: no chest pain

Respiratory: no shortness of breath

Musculoskeletal: pain in hands and feet

Neurological: no numbness

Eyes: negative

ENMT: negative

GI: some reflux with tomato based foods, which are avoided

GU: negative

Psych: negative

History

Past history includes vitamin D deficiency. Right hip replacement in 2008. Allergic to sulfa drugs.

Family history: father and sister also had RA

Social history: does not smoke or drink. Lives independently. Retired

Exam

General: well-developed white woman in no acute distress

Eyes: PERRLA/EOM; conjunctiva and sclera clear

ENMT: mucous membranes pink and moist

Cardiovascular: RRR

Respiratory: clear bilaterally to auscultation

GI: abdomen soft, non-tender, positive bowel sounds, no organomegaly

Skin: no rashes or lesions

Musculoskeletal: no active synovitis. Diffuse subluxations in wrists, hands, ankles, and toes.

Neuro: grossly intact

Psych: alert and oriented × 3, normal mood and affect

Medical decision making

Diagnosis: rheumatoid arthritis with no active disease. Patient's disease is "burnt out". Effects of the disease are evident though with obvious deformities and decreased function.

Data reviewed
None

Data ordered
Labs: CBC, ESR, AST, ALT, Cr

Treatment plan
We'll see Mary back in 6 months for a re-check. She should continue OTC pain relievers as needed.

Note 3

ENT Clinic new patient template

CC: Hemangioma

HPI
3-year-old white female presents with mother for facial hemangioma at base of right nasal fold. Present since birth, has not increased in size or changed visually. Spongy quality. Mother concerned that it obstructs the child's breathing. Does not itch or bleed spontaneously.

ROS
No fever or chills. No other respiratory issues besides breathing concern. No other vascular abnormalities noted by mother. Child is usually happy and easy-going.

History
Patient has no allergies

Exam
Constitutional: 3-year-old child is playing quietly in the exam room on entry. Sat in mother's arms willingly during exam.

Eyes: normal

Head: normocephalic, no step-offs or abnormalities

ENMT: TMs normal, outer ears normal; mucous membranes moist; throat normal; nares normal; right nare partially obstructed by hemangioma

Skin: no abnormalities noted on patient's arms, legs, or trunk; on face, 1.5 cm hemangioma partially obstructs patient's right nare. Appears to move gently with breath. Surrounding skin normal.

Medical decision making
Diagnosis: facial hemangioma

Data
None

Treatment plan
Will schedule the patient for surgery to remove hemangioma. Due to patient age and potential for complication of vascularization, will remove under general anesthesia.

Note 4

CC: Ear ache

HPI
Patient is well-known to the practice. Presents today with two-day history of right ear pain. Severe enough that it causes the child to cry.

ROS
Mother reports low-grade fever, no nasal drainage, cough

Exam
Constitutional: vital signs stable, temp low-grade fever

Eyes: clear.

ENMT: right tympanic membrane is bulging, injected, red

Continued

Note 4—cont'd

Diagnosis
Otitis media

Data
None

Plan
Amoxicillin by mouth, twice daily for 10 days

Note 5

Internal medicine clinic

CC: Follow-up hypertension

HPI
Patient has been compliant with medication, diet, and exercise. As a result patient has been losing weight, which will benefit his hypertension.

ROS
No chest pain

Exam
Blood pressure today is 133/80, which is much improved from his last visit
Lungs clear to auscultation
Heart regular

Diagnosis
1. Hypertension, improving
2. Obesity, improving

Data
Labs are normal

Plan
Continue ACE I, diet, and exercise. Return in 6 months for check-up.

Note 6

Pediatric endocrine clinic

CC: Thyroiditis

HPI
We had the pleasure of seeing the patient today, a 17-year-old, who we follow annually for Hashimoto thyroiditis and hypothyroidism, diagnosed when she was 8 years old. She has been doing well since we saw her a year ago. Patient has had trouble being compliant in taking her Synthroid without prompting from her parents. Occasionally misses a dose if not reminded. She has experienced some occasional diarrhea and mild cold/heat intolerance. Patient is concerned regarding recent burning sensation with urination.

Note 6—cont'd

ROS

Constitutional: no fever

GI: no diarrhea, no vomiting

GU: recent burning sensation with urination

Neurological: no weakness

Respiratory: no shortness of breath

Cardiovascular: no chest pain

Ears: no hearing difficulty

Endocrine: no polyuria, no polydipsia, mild heat/cold intolerance

History
Past: history of urinary tract infections

Exam
General: vital signs stable, overweight

HEENT: normal

Neck: supple. Thyroid mildly enlarged.

Lungs: clear

Heart: regular rate and rhythm

Abdomen: soft, positive bowel signs

Psych: alert and oriented, appropriate affect

Data
Labs: TSH slightly elevated; urinalysis positive

Diagnosis
Hashimoto thyroiditis, not improving
Urinary tract infection, new

Plan
Discussed with patient at length the importance of taking her medication regularly and the risks involved with non-compliance. Prescribed Keflex to treat UTI. Should have UTI re-checked in 10 days or so with primary care.

Note 7

Observation admit by cardiology

CC: Chest pain

HPI
Patient was admitted to observation from the emergency department with a 2-hour history of stabbing chest pain. Two sublingual nitros had not reduced the pain, currently at 9/10. The patient ate dinner 3 hours prior to presentation at ED.

ROS
Constitutional: no fever, no chills

Continued

Note 7—cont'd

Eyes: no diplopia

ENMT: no pain with swallowing

GI: no indigestion, no spicy or acidic foods at dinner

GU: negative

Musculoskeletal: negative

Cardiovascular: chest pain

Respiratory: some shortness of breath, secondary to chest pain

Integumentary: feels sweaty

Neurological: no dizziness

History
Coronary atherosclerosis
Family history of cardiac disease in father, uncle, and brother

Social history: does not smoke, 4 drinks × week, denies recreational drugs

Exam
Constitutional: patient is a 53-year-old white obese male in moderate distress

Eyes: normal

HEENT: normal

Cardiovascular: RRR, no murmurs, no rubs, no gallops; pulses normal in extremities x4; positive carotid pulse

Skin: diaphoretic

Musculoskeletal: no increased chest pain on chest wall palpation

Abdomen: no epigastric tenderness

Assessment and plan
Unstable angina, R/O MI. Order labs, cardiac catheterization.

Note 8

Hospitalist service note

CC: Dehydration

HPI
43-year-old male was admitted to observation with dehydration following extended environmental exposure to heat and sun without adequate water during a longer than expected recreational hike. Patient is also reporting symptoms of mild heat exhaustion. The patient tried to resolve symptoms by drinking an excess of water following the hike, but was not able to keep it down.

ROS
Constitutional: no recent weight change

Eyes: no vision changes

ENMT: positive dry mouth

Cardiac: feels like his heart is pounding.

Respiratory: no shortness of breath

Note 8—cont'd

GI: Unable to take any water PO as it results in vomiting

GU: Reports very yellow urine

Musculoskeletal: mild muscle cramping

Neurological: feels "woozy" and lightheaded when standing

Endocrine: no polyuria, no polydipsia

Psychological: no unusual ideation, no anxiety or depression

PFSH

Past history: no hypertension, no diabetes, no history of dehydration

Family history: no heart disease

Social history: patient enjoys recreational hiking with moderately good fitness

Exam

Constitutional: middle-aged appearing man in no acute distress; pulse is slightly elevated, hypotensive, low-grade fever

Eyes: clear

ENT: mucous membranes moist

Cardiovascular: RRR, no rubs, no murmurs, no gallops

Respiratory: clear to auscultation bilaterally, slightly elevated respiration

GI: soft, non-tender, no organomegaly

GU: normal external genitalia

Musculoskeletal: full ROM in extremities, soreness and mild pain with movement

Integumentary: skin is pale, clammy to the touch.

Psychological: moderately alert; oriented to person, place, and time

Assessment and plan

Patient has moderate dehydration. Will hold in observation to determine whether short-term treatment is effective. Concern for kidney function. Push IV fluids. PO clear liquids when tolerated. Monitor urine output.

Note 9

Pulmonary service—Observation admit note

CC: Cough

HPI

Patient presented to the Emergency Department with an unresolvable cough for 24 hours. The patient has a long history of asthma, chronic bronchitis, and other respiratory ailments. The patient reports the cough is the worst it has ever been. Patient also reports significant shortness of breath with mild activity. It feels like the patient just can't get a full breath.

ROS

Constitutional: no fever, no chills

Respiratory: see HPI

Cardiovascular: no chest pain

Continued

Note 9—cont'd

GI: negative

Neurological: negative
All others negative

PFSH

Past history: asthma, environmental allergies, chronic bronchitis. ALLERGIC TO SULFA

Family history: no associated family history

Social history: 20-year smoking history 1-2 packs/day

Exam
Constitutional: patient appears exhausted and slightly diaphoretic. Patient frequently must stop the exam for an extended coughing bout. VSS

HEENT: normal

Cardiovascular: RRR

Respiratory: wheezes present bilaterally. Obvious retractions, Barrel-chest present. Pursed-lip breathing.

Integumentary: mildly cyanotic

Psychological: alert and oriented ×3, tearful

Assessment and plan
Probable COPD severely exacerbated by asthma and long-term tobacco use. Counseled the patient concerning tobacco cessation, but patient is reluctant.
Ordered spirometry, labs, CT to determine diagnosis.
Initiate albuterol treatments immediately. Prednisone, Singular ordered.
Monitor oximetry. Consider full admission if patient does not respond to treatment.

Note 10

Cardiology note

CC: Chest pain obs day 2

HPI
[Patient was admitted to observation from the emergency department with a 2 hour history of stabbing chest pain. Two sublingual nitros had not reduced the pain, currently at 9/10. The patient ate dinner 3 hours prior to presentation at ED.] Since yesterday, patient reports chest pain is well-controlled 2 or 3/10. No associated symptoms.

ROS
Eyes: no diplopia

ENMT: no pain with swallowing

GI: no indigestion

GU: negative

Respiratory: shortness of breath has resolved with pain control and rest

Integumentary: sweating resolved

Neurological: no dizziness

Exam
Eyes: normal

Note 10—cont'd

HEENT: normal

Cardiovascular: RRR, no murmurs, no rubs, no gallops; pulses normal in extremities x4; positive carotid pulse

Skin: dry

Musculoskeletal: no increased chest pain on chest wall palpation

Abdomen: No epigastric tenderness

Assessment and plan
Cardiac cath revealed blocked vessel, which was treated with stent. Angina is resolving. Will hold patient until tomorrow, continuing to monitor underlying heart disease and related symptoms.

Note 11

Hospitalist service note

CC: Dehydration

HPI
43-year-old male was admitted to observation yesterday with dehydration following extended environmental exposure. Patient is feeling much better this morning following IV hydration. Reports feeling less warm, less shaky.

Exam
Constitutional: vital signs look better. Fever is reduced, blood pressure improved, pulse normal

Integumentary: skin is pinker than yesterday, dry

Assessment and plan
Patient has improving moderate dehydration. Will hold in observation to determine whether short-term treatment is effective. Concern for kidney function. Push IV fluids. PO clear liquids when tolerated. Monitor urine output.

Note 12

Pulmonary service—obs day 2

CC: Cough

HPI
Overnight patient reports improvement with shortness of breath

ROS
Constitutional: no fever, no chills

Respiratory: See HPI

Cardiovascular: no chest pain

Exam
Constitutional: patient appears stable today

Respiratory: wheezes present bilaterally

Assessment and plan
COPD severely exacerbated by asthma and long-term tobacco use. COPD improving today.
Continue prescription medications as ordered. Monitor oximetry. Will continue to monitor.

Note 13

Initial admission to psychiatric service

CC: Suicidal ideation

HPI

(Some history was collected from the patient's parents.) 16-year-old male with recent suicidal ideations × 2 months. Parents found extensive suicide method information on the patient's computer. Patient has expressed hopelessness to his parents and they have noticed his appetite is reduced. Patient confirms. He states he feels the worst he ever has.

ROS

Constitutional: recent weight loss

Eyes: no vision changes

Psychological: patient reports feelings of hopelessness
All others negative.

History

Past history: no illnesses, no surgeries, no known drug allergies

Family history: father diagnosed with moderate depression

Social history: parents note suspicion of recreational drug use. Patient denies alcohol, tobacco, drugs. Patient is a junior in high school, but has recently stopped attending classes regularly.

Exam
HEENT: normal

Cardiovascular: RRR

Respiratory: clear to auscultation bilaterally

GI: no guarding, no rebound, no tenderness, positive bowel sounds

Musculoskeletal: strength and coordination normal

Neurological: sensation, reflexes normal

Immunological: no cervical lymphadenopathy

Psychological: patient is alert, oriented ×3, tearful. We discussed his situation at length.

Assessment and plan
Qualitative labs negative.
Will complete psychiatric diagnostic examination tomorrow if patient is feeling better.
Xanax ordered.
Patient to remain under suicide watch on inpatient ward.

Note 14

Pediatric inpatient admission

CC: Dysphagia

HPI

Patient has a 2-week history of sore throat. Strep test was negative at Primary Care office, which recommended conservative management including salt water gargles. Patient has worsened and now complains of dysphagia for 2 days. He also reports a fever. The swallowing is bad enough that the patient is reluctant to swallow, instead expectorating.

Note 14—cont'd

ROS

Constitutional: fever

Eyes: negative

ENMT: negative other than HPI

Cardiovascular: negative

Respiratory: negative

GI: negative

GU: negative

Musculoskeletal: maybe a little achy

Neurological: negative

Psychological: negative

History

Patient history: history of strep throat. No known drug allergies

Family history: no family history of throat problems

Social history: has not been around anyone with reported mononucleosis. Attends school regularly.

Exam

Constitutional: patient appears in mild distress. Lean, 15-year-old male.

Eyes: clear

ENMT: throat is red, swollen, tonsils are enlarged and showing signs of necrosis and tonsilloliths. Airway is not obstructed.

Immunological: cervical nodes are mildly enlarged

Cardiovascular: RRR

Respiratory: clear

GI: Soft non-tender, no guarding, no rebound

Psychological: alert and oriented ×3

Musculoskeletal: normal

Neurological: grossly normal

Assessment and plan

Strep and mono labs negative. Viral acute tonsillitis. Patient scheduled for tonsillectomy tomorrow.

Note 15

Admit note

CC: Pneumonia

HPI

Patient is a 74-year-old male with diagnosed pneumonia. Symptoms began about 10 days ago including productive cough, fever, fatigue, and chills. The patient reports symptoms as 7/10. Patient tried a number of over-the-counter medications before seeking treatment.

ROS

See HPI

Continued

Note 15—cont'd

History

Past history: pneumonia 5 years ago

Social history: no tobacco

Exam

Constitutional: fever. Oxygen sats 92% on room air. 100% on nasal cannula. Cervical lymph nodes mildly swollen.

Respiratory: inspirations show mild distress. On percussion, chest is dull. Decreased air intake. Mild wheezes. No rales. Rust colored sputum.

Psychological: Alert and oriented ×3

Assessment and plan

Chest x-ray positive for pneumonia. Likely bacterial pneumonia, but have sent sputum to lab to see if anything grows out. Antibiotics ordered.

Note 16

Inpatient day 2

CC: Fever

HPI

Mother reports patient does not feel warm to the touch and is happy and more responsive today

ROS

No subjective fever

Exam

Constitutional: vital signs stable; temp 99.7; awake and in no acute distress

Psychological: responsive, happy, alert to surroundings; smiles spontaneously

Diagnosis

Fever improving

Data

Lab cultures negative to date

Plan

Continue ampicillin 110 mg IV q 6 hr; gentamycin 10 mg IV q 8 hr

Note 17

Admit note

CC: Pneumonia

HPI

Patient is improved overnight. Reports breathing easier.

Exam

Constitutional fever. Oxygen sats 92% on room air. 100% on nasal cannula. Elevated BP—new onset. Cervical lymph nodes mildly swollen.

Note 17—cont'd

Respiratory: inspirations show mild distress. On percussion, chest is dull. Decreased air intake. Mild wheezes. no rales. Sputum light rust.

Assessment and plan
1. Cultures showed bacterial pneumonia. Patient is clinically stable. Continue antibiotic plan.
2. Moderate hypertension. Start Lasix.

Note 18

Nephrology progress note

CC: Hypertension

HPI
Patient is inpatient stay day 2. Post-kidney transplant ×6 months. Patient measured high blood pressures at home for 4 days. Patient also reports mild leg swelling and decreased urine output.

ROS
Constitutional: patient feels lethargic

Cardiovascular: subjective high blood pressures measured at home, leg swelling

GU: decreased urine output

Exam
Constitutional: elevated BP; moderate fever

Cardiovascular: mild lower extremity edema; RRR

Respiratory: clear to auscultation bilaterally; slightly increased respirations

GI: abdomen is slightly distended, suspect fluid

Assessment and plan
1. Elevated blood pressure (worsening)
2. Fluid retention (worsening)
Ordering labs, Pelvic CT, lower extremity Doppler ultrasound. Discussed the patient's case with attending transplant surgeon.
Patient has probable transplant rejection. Will continue monitoring symptoms and adjust medications.

Note 19

Hospitalist obs admit note time: 0210

CC: Facial pain

HPI
Patient was admitted from the ED where he presenting immediately following an altercation. Patient admitted to intoxication prior to the altercation. Patient notes acute throbbing pain in his central face. He reports being hit with fists, no other implements. Pain is 6/10. Patient also reports swallowing blood. Does not think he lost any teeth.

ROS
See HPI. All others negative.

Continued

Note 19—cont'd

History

Past history: no prior surgeries or hospitalizations. Broken nose ×2 years ago. No known drug allergies.

Family history: reports no bleeding disorders

Social history: 8-12 alcoholic drinks on weekend nights

Exam

Constitutional: 23-year-old white male in mild distress. Vitals stable.

Eyes: reddened conjunctiva

Ears: normal

Nose: swollen, obvious fracture, nares swollen, packed with tamponade

Mouth: dentition intact; no visible injury

Cardiovascular: RRR

Respiratory: CTAB

Musculoskeletal: Other than nasal bone fracture, head appears normocephalic, atraumatic, no step-offs. Extremities normal.

GI: abdomen is soft, non-tender, no guarding, no rebound, positive bowel sounds

GU: normal external male genitalia

Skin: face mildly abraded

Neurological: patient is drowsy but arousable. Glasgow scale 13

Assessment and plan

Head CT shows fractured nasal bone as well as maxillary hairline fracture. Concerned regarding patient's neurologic status. Ordered repeat CT to rule out intracranial hematoma. Will monitor patient's neurologic status through the day and stabilize fractures.

Hospitalist observation discharge note Time: 1830

Patient was admitted early this morning for observation following a fistfight. Patient initially had reduced consciousness that resolved throughout the day. Fractures are stable. Hemodynamically stable. CT was negative. Patient discharged with head trauma instructions and follow-up appointment with surgeon to correct nasal fracture.

Note 20

Daily progress note

CC: Anal pain

HPI

Patient is a 27-year-old female who vaginally delivered a healthy child 4 weeks ago. Since then, the patient has experienced significant constipation. Last night, after straining and ultimately passing a small amount of hard stool, the patient experienced severe anal pain reported as 9/10. She noted blood on tissue, but not in the toilet. No associated vaginal pain. Patient called our nurse line, which directed her to the hospital where we admitted her to assess the complaint.

ROS

Constitutional: no fevers

GI: constipation

GU: no discharge

All others negative

Note 20—cont'd

History
Past history: vaginal delivery × 4 weeks

Family history: no history of colon ca or other lower GI cancers

Social history: no tobacco; 1 drink daily; no recreational drugs

Exam
Constitutional: patient is tearful and curled on her side. Vital signs stable.

Cardiovascular: RRR

Respiratory: CTAB

GI: abdomen is moderately tender, obvious retained stool; reduced bowel sounds; rectal exam is difficult due to pain. Will defer until pain medication is administered.

GU: normal post-delivery external genitalia. No evidence of trauma or complication.

Musculoskeletal: normal

Integumentary: normal

Neurological: grossly normal

Assessment and plan
Patient has suspected anal fissure. Will re-examine after patient's pain is controlled. Ordered IV morphine.

Interim note
Patient reports pain is controlled. On exam patient has anal fissure. Plan is to soften stools, ensure constipation is cleared.

Discharge note
Patient was discharged late this afternoon following constipation treatment. Sent home with instructions to promote healthy bowel movements and manage fissure. Hydrocodone script.

Note 21

This note is very similar to Note 20 with one significant difference that affects the E&M level. Audit the note carefully and note the difference one piece of information makes.

Daily progress note

CC: Anal pain

HPI
Patient is a 27-year-old female who vaginally delivered a healthy child 4 weeks ago. Since then, the patient has experienced significant constipation. Last night, after straining and ultimately passing a small amount of hard stool, the patient experienced severe anal pain reported as 9/10. She noted blood on tissue, but not in the toilet. No associated vaginal pain. Patient called our nurse line, which directed her to the hospital where we admitted her to assess the complaint.

ROS
Constitutional: no fevers

GI: constipation

GU: no discharge
All others negative

History
Past history: vaginal delivery × 4 weeks

Social history: no tobacco; 1 drink daily; no recreational drugs

Continued

Note 21—cont'd

Exam

Constitutional: patient is tearful and curled on her side. Vital signs stable.

Cardiovascular: RRR

Respiratory: CTAB

GI: Abdomen is moderately tender, obvious retained stool; reduced bowel sounds; rectal exam is difficult due to pain. Will defer until pain medication is administered.

GU: Normal post-delivery external genitalia. No evidence of trauma or complication.

Musculoskeletal: normal

Integumentary: normal

Neurological: grossly normal

Assessment and plan

Patient has suspected anal fissure. Will re-examine after patient's pain is controlled. Ordered IV morphine.

Interim note

Patient reports pain is controlled. On exam patient has anal fissure. Plan is to soften stools, ensure constipation is cleared.

Discharge note

Patient was discharged late this afternoon following constipation treatment. Sent home with instructions to promote healthy bowel movements and manage fissure. Hydrocodone script.

Note 22

November 17, 2010
Re: Jane Smith
Dear Dr. Jones,
Thank you for asking me to see your patient, Jane Smith, to assess her skin condition. Ms. Smith presented with a 4-month history of a rash. The rash itches. It is itchy enough that it wakes Ms. Smith from sleep. The rash began on her lower legs and has spread to her entire legs, trunk, and arms. The patient has tried a number of over the counter lotions and creams to soothe her skin.

ROS

Constitutional: sleep disturbed by itching. No fevers.

Eyes: itchy and watery secondary to environmental allergies

Nose: some sneezing and post-nasal drip

Skin: see HPI

History

Past history: patient has environmental allergies moderately controlled by Allegra with breakthrough symptoms when allergens are high.

Exam

Constitutional: vital signs stable

Eyes: moderately reddened. Pupils equal, round, reactive to light and accommodation.

ENMT: mucous membranes moist

Cardiovascular: RRR

Note 22—cont'd

Respiratory: CTAB

Skin: lower extremity skin is raw and broken from scratching. Diffuse blistering. No signs of infection. Trunk and upper extremities show red rash, some swelling and rawness. Thickened skin on hips from chronic inflammation. Hands, feet, and head are clear.

Assessment and plan
Ms. Smith is unfortunately suffering from atopic dermatitis. We gave her handouts on home care for this condition. Benadryl can be taken at bedtime to ease nighttime itching. Script written for steroid cream to apply twice a day. She should return to clinic in 2 weeks, sooner if symptoms persist.
Again, thank you for allowing me to see Ms. Smith.

Note 23

I was asked to see the patient by Dr. Johnson to assess a bruise. Patient reports a persistent bruise just below the knee present for 1 month. Patient reports repeatedly hitting her leg on entering the bathtub. On exam, there is no significant vascular damage at the injury site. Patient should avoid hitting the leg. She can apply a warm cloth or heat pack to the area several times a day to speed healing. Patient should seek immediate help if there is any extreme pain or swelling at the site.
cc: Dr. Johnson

Note 24

[Note is entered in a shared medical record of a multi-specialty practice.]

ENT clinic note

CC: Ear ache

HPI
Patient is a 3-year-old charming boy that Dr. Kim asked me to see regarding treatment for chronic otitis media. The patient has experienced ear infections since approximately 6 months of age.

ROS
Constitutional: no current fever

Ear: no current pain

Exam
Constitutional: patient is a pleasant boy who appears in no acute distress

Ear: tympanic membrane shows evidence of chronic inflammation

Neck: no cervical lymphadenopathy

Assessment and plan
Patient has chronic otitis media. Will schedule patient for tympanostomy.

Note 25

Orthopedic inpatient consult service

Endocrine asked us to see the patient today concerning right foot gangrene.

HPI
The patient has developed gangrene of the right foot in the context of peripheral vascular disease secondary to diabetes type II.

ROS
No pain in the foot, though it had been extremely painful for a short time. Left foot no pain.

Past history
Diabetic

Exam
Constitutional: vital signs stable with low grade fever.

Musculoskeletal: gangrenous right foot involving great toe, 2nd and 3rd toes, distal third of associated metatarsal region.

Integumentary: skin ranges from blue to black. Obvious foul smell.

Neurological: not painful to the touch or pin prick.

Assessment and plan
Patient will be taken to OR for mid-foot amputation emergently to prevent further spread of gangrene.

Note 26

[Note is entered in the shared inpatient record.]

Endocrine note

CC: High glucose levels

Consulting physician: Dr. Singh

HPI
We were consulted to see the patient and determine whether she has developed DM II. Patient is admitted for total hip replacement. In the course of her pre-operative preparations last week, she was found to have a high random glucose level. Patient reports increased thirst and urination for 6 months. Patient has never been diagnosed with diabetes and has not made any dietary changes to lower her risk of diabetes.

ROS
Constitutional: no fevers

Eyes: no blurred vision

ENMT: no dry mouth

Cardiovascular: no chest pain

Respiratory: no shortness of breath

Endocrine: positive for polydipsia and polyuria × 6 months

History
Past history: total right hip replacement

Family history: sister with DM II

Exam
Constitutional: vital signs stable

HEENT: normal

Note 26—cont'd

Cardiovascular: RRR

Respiratory: CTAB

GI: soft, non-tender, no guarding, no rebound, positive bowel sounds

GU: no flank pain over kidneys

Neurological: grossly normal

Psychological: Alert and oriented × 3

Lymphatic: No cervical or inguinal lymphadenopathy

Assessment and plan
Abnormal glucose levels. Will order patient's first A1C. Diabetic diet ordered preemptively. Will continue to follow while admitted.

Note 27

[Note is entered in shared inpatient medical record]

Gastroenterology consult service

Requesting Physician: Dr. Nguyen

CC: Hyperemesis

HPI
Patient admitted with alcoholic cirrhosis complicated by ascites now has 12-hour history of emesis. Patient notes this is the first time he has experienced this level of emesis. This is the worst emesis he has ever had. Patient notes emesis quality is that of coffee grounds. Patient is vomiting every few hours.

ROS
Constitutional: patient feels clammy and weak

GI: See HPI

All others negative

Exam
Constitutional: patient is a 63-year-old white male who is pale and tearful on presentation

Eyes: jaundiced

ENMT: within normal limits

Cardiovascular: slightly tachycardic

Respiratory: breaths sounds are shallow and increased

GI: patient's abdomen is distended by ascites with positive fluid wave.

Integumentary: jaundiced

Neurological: grossly normal

Psychiatric: alert and oriented × 3, tearful, expresses depressed feelings at his medical conditions

Assessment and plan
Patient has significant coffee ground emesis. Called the lab to schedule urgent upper endoscopy. Suspect slow GI bleed secondary to alcoholic cirrhosis.

Note 28

CC: Pain

HPI

33-year-old African-American female presents to the ED with constant abdominal pain, which has been present for 2 days. The pain has a burning and cramping quality. On a pain scale the patient reports 8/10. The patient cannot identify anything that makes the pain worse or that occurred when the pain began. The patient has tried a variety of home remedies that have not relieved the pain. Patient is not experiencing nausea, vomiting, constipation, or hematemesis.

ROS

GI: see HPI

All others negative

PFSH

Past history: HTN, morbidly obese, no known drug allergies

Family history: no AAA or heart disease

Social history: no tobacco, social alcohol, no recreational drugs

Exam

Constitutional: moderately elevated blood pressure, morbidly obese, moderate distress

Eyes: normal

Cardiovascular: regular rate and rhythm; neck and extremity pulses normal

Respiratory: normal breath sounds

Abdomen: no scars, positive bowel sounds, positive Murphy's sign, aorta normal, no guarding, no rebound

GU: external genitalia normal

Musculoskeletal: normal strength and tone

Neurological: grossly normal

Psychiatric: normal affect, alert and oriented

Medical decision making
Data reviewed

Lab: positive urine dip pregnancy

Diagnosis

Abdominal pain, possible ectopic pregnancy

Plan

Admit to observation, OB consulted

Note 29

CC: Knee pain

HPI

Patient presents to ED post pedestrian vs. car collision last night. Patient was pedestrian walking in street. Primary concern is right knee pain. Pain is 8/10. Pain occurs at rest and with movement. Patient describes the pain as sharp. No other pain, no bleeding, no reported deformity, no other symptoms.

Note 29—cont'd

ROS
Musculoskeletal no pain other than noted in HPI. No fever, no chills, no vision problems, no nasal discharge, no chest pain, no shortness of breath, no abdominal pain, no dysuria, no rashes, no loss of consciousness, no depression or anxiety, no unusual bruising.

PFSH
No prior surgeries. No known drug allergies. No family hx of arthritis. Positive tobacco. Positive alcohol. Denies recreational drugs.

Exam
40-year-old BM in mild distress. VS normal except increased heart rate. Head normocephalic, no crepitus, no step-offs. Eyes normal. Mucous membranes pink and moist. Neck supple. Heart normal on auscultation. Breath sounds normal bilaterally. Abdomen appears normal, positive bowel sounds, soft, no guarding. Right knee limited range of motion, painful to touch. Alert and oriented. Grossly normal neurologically.

Data
Lab panel normal
Knee x-ray (personally reviewed film) shows proximal tibial fracture

Plan
Pain treated tonight with IV morphine, well controlled on discharge. Knee placed in brace. Follow-up in ortho clinic next week.

Note 30

CC: Dizzy

Subjective: 75-year-old patient presents with history of dizziness since 6:00 am this morning. Patient feels like the "room is spinning around me". The dizziness ebbs and flows but has not completely resolved. Patient is also experiencing unstable feeling, mild nausea, and a headache. Laying down makes the feeling worse. ROS is otherwise negative. History of controlled hypertension. No family history of stroke. Patient does not smoke.

Objective: vital signs stable. WF in no moderate distress. Pupils equal and round, reactive to light, mild nystagmus. Mucous membranes moist. Neck supple. Heart regular rate and rhythm. Negative positional hypotension. Breath sounds normal. Positive bowel sounds. Full range of motion in all extremities. No rashes. Alert and oriented. Patient is unable to walk a line without one or two hand support. Able to complete finger-to-nose. Hearing normal.

Assessment and plan: lab panel normal. CT head normal. Patient is experiencing vertigo and headache, but needs further testing to determine definitive diagnosis. Responded well to IV meds. Discharged home with neurology appointment.

Note 31

CC: Late effects of stroke

HPI
Patient experienced a stroke 14 days ago resulting in left-sided hemiplegia. Patient is minimally communicative but denied any other significant symptoms. Admitted to long-term skilled nursing care.

Continued

Note 31—cont'd

ROS
Patient denies significant musculoskeletal pain and no vision deficits

PFSH
Patient's spouse confirmed PFSH

Past history: hypertension

Social history: no tobacco, no drugs, previously a social drinker, a couple of drinks a week

Exam
Constitutional: patient appears to be resting comfortably in bed

Eyes: normal

ENMT: mucous membranes clear

Cardiovascular: RRR

Respiratory: CTAB

GI: patient has significant trouble swallowing and is receiving parenteral nutrition. Bowel sounds are present. No tenderness.

Musculoskeletal: left-side arm and leg with minimal movement, though the patient is able to make small movements. Right-side adequate function.

Neurological: absent grasp left-side; patient is able to vocalize, but has significant difficultly forming words and currently chooses not to attempt.

Psychiatric: alert and oriented × 3. Depressed mood.

Assessment
1. Hemiplegia secondary to stroke
2. Dysphagia
3. Dysphasia
4. Depression

Plan
Hemiplegia is likely chronic. Will initiate PT and OT to maximize function with goals including eating soft foods and improving speech. Psych consult to monitor depression and discuss family support.

Note 32

CC: Late effects of stroke

HPI
Patient experienced a stroke 14 days ago resulting in left-sided hemiplegia. Patient is minimally communicative but denied any other significant symptoms. Admitted to long-term skilled nursing care.

ROS
Patient denies significant musculoskeletal pain and no vision deficits. AON

PFSH
Patient's spouse confirmed PFSH.

Past history: hypertension

Family history: parents deceased, father of stroke.

Social history: no tobacco, no drugs, previously a social drinker, a couple of drinks a week.

Note 32—cont'd

Exam

Constitutional: patient appears to be resting comfortably in bed

Eyes: normal

ENMT: mucous membranes clear

Cardiovascular: RRR

Respiratory: CTAB

GI: patient has significant trouble swallowing and is receiving parenteral nutrition. Bowel sounds are present. No tenderness.

Musculoskeletal: left-side arm and leg with minimal movement, though the patient is able to make small movements. Right-side adequate function.

Neurological: absent grasp left-side; patient is able to vocalize, but has significant difficultly forming words and currently chooses not to attempt.

Psychiatric: alert and oriented × 3. Depressed mood.

Assessment

1. Hemiplegia secondary to stroke
2. Dysphagia
3. Dysphasia
4. Depression

Plan

Hemiplegia is likely chronic. Will initiate PT and OT to maximize function with goals including eating soft foods and improving speech. Psych consult to monitor depression and discuss family support.

Note 33

CC: Late effects of stroke

HPI

Patient experienced a stroke 14 days ago resulting in left-sided hemiplegia. Patient is not communicative; spouse denies any other significant symptoms. Admitted to long-term skilled nursing care.

ROS

Spouse denies significant musculoskeletal pain and no vision deficits

PFSH

Spouse confirmed PFSH

Past history: hypertension

Family history: parents deceased, father of stroke

Social history: 2 pack/day tobacco, no drugs, previously a social drinker, a couple of drinks a week

Exam

Constitutional: patient appears to be resting comfortably in bed

Eyes: normal

ENMT: mucous membranes clear

Cardiovascular: RRR

Respiratory: wheezes noted bilaterally; mass in right lobe noted during hospital admission

Continued

Note 33—cont'd

GI: Patient has significant trouble swallowing and is receiving parenteral nutrition. Bowel sounds are present. No tenderness.

Musculoskeletal: left-side arm and leg with minimal movement, though the patient is able to make small movements. Right-side adequate function.

Neurological: absent grasp left-side; patient is able to vocalize, but has significant difficultly forming words and currently chooses not to attempt.

Psychiatric: alert and oriented × 3. Depressed mood.

Assessment
1. Hemiplegia secondary to stroke
2. Dysphagia
3. Dysphasia
4. Depression
5. Lung mass

Plan
Hemiplegia is likely chronic. With history or hypertension and smoking, patient is at significant risk for future strokes. Will initiate PT and OT to maximize function with goals including eating soft foods and improving speech. Psych consult to monitor depression and discuss family support. Ordered chest CT to evaluate chest mass.

Note 34

CC: Runny nose

HPI
6-year-old patient is new to our practice and presents with her parents today concerned with chronic runny nose, sneezing, itchy eyes, and cough × 1 year. Patient's symptoms are worse in the spring and fall. Parents suspect environmental allergies and would like the patient evaluated.

ROS
See HPI. Parents also report some itchy skin. No lymph node enlargement.

PFSH
No hospitalizations, no surgeries. Mother is allergic to multiple environmental allergens as well as severe allergy to tree nuts.

Exam
Constitutional: patient is a pleasant young girl in no apparent distress

Eyes: are moderately injected and watery

Nose: nares are reddened and inflamed, post-nasal drip present

Ears: normal

Mouth: moist, good dentition

Throat: unaffected, tonsils normal

Neck: no lymphadenopathy

Assessment and plan
Patient is experiencing typical allergic symptoms. Instructed parents on administering Benadryl and maintaining environmental hygiene to reduce symptoms. Scheduled consultation with an allergist.

■ INTERMEDIATE

You may need to review medical information in order to appropriately code these notes.

Note 35

HPI
New patient comes to see us in clinic today regarding RUQ pain, especially after eating a fatty meal. Patient describes the pain as dull and constant when it is present. Patient has been experiencing the pain for 1 week.

ROS
No recent weight gain/loss. No chest pain. No shortness of breath. GI postprandial pain. GU no urinary symptoms. No chest wall pain.

PFSH
Med list includes daily Zyrtec and Benadryl. Occasional Tums. No tobacco, no illicits, 2 drinks a couple of times a week.

Exam
Patient is a pleasant, obese woman in no current distress. Moderately elevated blood pressure, otherwise VSS. RRR. CTAB. Positive Murphy's sign. No LUQ, RLQ or LLQ tenderness. Positive bowel sounds. No guarding. No rebound. No jaundice.

Tests
CBC normal. Ultrasound positive for gallbladder stones per report.

Assessment
Cholecystitis

Plan
Scheduled the patient for laparoscopic cholecystectomy with grams in 10 days. Instructed the patient on a gallbladder diet until then.

Note 36

HPI
Patient is seen today in derm clinic for the first time with concern regarding a lesion located in the left axillar crease. Patient is worried because the lesion has been growing over the past year and is now fleshy and protruding. Lesion is not painful or itchy, does not bleed or catch on clothing.

ROS
See HPI. Patient has not noted other lesions.

Exam
VSS. Lesion is light brown with regular margins.

Assessment
Skin tag

Plan
Assured the patient that this is a benign lesion, and that skin tags will grow, but are not malignant. Offered to remove the skin tag but discussed that this would probably not be covered by insurance. Patient decided to wait on removal. Encouraged the patient in checking her skin for lesions and discussed the characteristics of suspicious lesions. We will see the patient back if removal is desired.

Note 37

CC: Acne

History
Patient returns today having started using prescription topical on upper body acne. Patient has been compliant in applying the medications as directed. Patient thinks it is helping and reports reduced breakouts and less inflammation.

Exam
Patient's skin does look improved.

Assessment and plan
Continue using topicals as prescribed for acne. Return in 6 months.

Note 38

Patient returns to endocrinology clinic today.

CC: Neuropathy

HPI
Patient reports experiencing increased diabetic related neuropathy for the past 3 months. Patient is not compliant with prescribed diet and exercise programs and has forgotten to bring in blood sugar journals today. Notes increased numbness and a small persistent blister.

ROS
See HPI. No weight changes. No chest pain. No SOB. AON.

PFSH
No recent hospitalizations. Family history of DM II. Lives alone in assisted living.

Exam
VSS

HEENT: normal

Card: RRR, pedal pulses reduced

Resp: CTAB

GI: no tenderness; bowel sounds positive

Musculoskeletal: full ROM

Neuro: Decreased sensation bilateral feet, ankle reflexes

Integument: hair absent on lower legs; blister on right foot has obviously been repeatedly rubbed
Psych alert and oriented times three

Tests
A1c 7.8

Assessment and plan
Increasing neuropathy—increase duloxetine to 60 mg twice daily; ordered EMG to determine extent
Blister—drained today with instructions for bandaging and preventing further blisters. Referred to shoe store that carries shoes that will be safer.
Uncontrolled Diabetes—Spent a long time talking about patient's barriers to compliance. Patient assured me of intent to be compliant going forward. Will see the patient back in 1 month for recheck.

Note 39

Hospitalist service note

History
43-year-old male was admitted to observation with dehydration following extended environmental exposure to heat and sun without adequate water during a longer than expected recreational hike. Patient is also reporting symptoms of mild heat exhaustion. The patient tried to resolve symptoms by drinking an excess of water following the hike, but was not able to keep it down.

ROS
No recent weight change, No vision changes, Positive dry mouth, Feels like his heart is pounding, no shortness of breath, unable to take any water po as it results in vomiting, reports very yellow urine, mild muscle cramping, feels woozy and lightheaded when standing, no polyuria, no polydipsia, no unusual ideation

PFSH
No hypertension, no diabetes, no history of dehydration, no heart disease, patient enjoys recreational hiking with moderately good fitness, no tobacco, no ETOH, no drugs

Exam
Middle-aged appearing man in no acute distress; pulse is slightly elevated, hypotensive, low-grade fever, eyes clear, mucous membranes moist; RRR, no rubs, no murmurs, no gallops; chest clear to auscultation bilaterally, slightly elevated respiration; abdomen soft, non-tender, no organomegaly; skin is pale, clammy to the touch; moderately alert; oriented times three

Assessment and plan
Patient has moderate dehydration. Will hold in observation to determine whether short-term treatment is effective. PO clear liquids when tolerated. Monitor urine output.

Note 40

Obs day 2

History
Patient suffered a blood clot at the femoral insertion site post heart cath yesterday. Patient was held in observation, started on heparin therapy. Patient is cheerful this morning, reporting reduced LE pain since last evening. No pain noted in other extremities.

Exam
VSS, slightly hypotensive. Reduced pedal pulse in affected leg, but improved from last night. Contralateral pulse normal. Capillary refill is reduced in affected leg. Leg continues to be cool on palpation and pale.

Assessment and plan
Acute arterial embolism. Continue heparin infusion. Surgical consult this am.

Note 41

History
8-year-old patient was admitted this morning following an acute asthma attack. Patient currently reports difficulty breathing, severity 9/10. Attack began approximately 4 hours ago. ED treatment was not effective in resolving the attack. Reports recent increase in attacks, increased need for rescue inhaler. Family has not recently moved into a new home or had any home changes including new pets, mold, leaks, air conditioning changes. Patient suffers from significant environmental allergies. Denies weight change, trouble sleeping, polyuria, polydipsia, cough, headache.

Continued

Note 41—cont'd

Exam
VSS, elevated heart rate. O_2 sats on room air 90%, 100% on cannula. Eyes normal. ENMT normal. No cervical lymphadenopathy. Card RRR. Resp significant wheezes bilaterally on expiration and inspiration, no crackling, no rhonchi, positive use of accessory muscles. Mild cyanosis.

Tests
Spirometry ordered. Requested copy of lab results from ED when complete. Discussed patient's past history of severe attacks with patient's primary care physician.

Assessment and plan
Status asthmaticus. IV magnesium sulfate. Albuterol treatments.

Note 42

History
Patient admitted from ED to plastic surgery service. 37-year-old patient was bicycling on a park path. A dog darted out in front of the patient, who applied the front tire brake instead of the rear brake. The bicycle stopped abruptly, throwing the patient forward over the handlebars, causing the patient to strike against pavement. Patient complains of throbbing, constant pain in her mid-face region, "under her nose," 10/10 severity. No pain reported in other body areas. Denies LOC at scene. Unable to complete additional history as the patient is tearful and sedated with pain medication.

Exam
37-year-old Asian female in moderate distress. Obvious mid-face deformity. Superficial scrapes on face. Skull is patent. No rhinorrhea or hemorrhage. No orbital deformity. No visual deficit. No otorrhea or hemorrhage. Dentition intact. Minor vestibule laceration. Lips intact. Palate is mobile. No throat trauma. Answers questions appropriately, but somnolent. Alert and oriented ×3. Cranial nerves II-XII normal. No cervical lymphadenopathy. Trachea midline.

Assessment and plan
CBC ordered. Neck plain films clear.
Likely Leforte II, but axial CT ordered for confirmation. Schedule surgery this afternoon. Continue morphine IV.

Note 43

Hospital day 1

CC: Urinary retention

History
Upon admission, 83-year-old male patient reports inability to pass urine x24 hours. Patient feels urgency, but unable to initiate stream. Patient does have BPH, which has caused problems urinating in the past. ROS is positive for sweating, increased pulse, and anxiety. AON. No tobacco/no ETOH. No fam hx of prostate ca. Hypertension controlled with ACE inhibitor.

Exam
83-year-old male in moderate distress. Hypertensive. Patient is sweating profusely. HEENT normal. Card RRR elevated pulse. Respirations increased. No GI tenderness, no guarding, no rebound. GU, normal external genitalia. Urinary catheter returned 1800 ml initially. Urine flowing normally. Neuro grossly normal. AAO×3.

Assessment and plan
Urinary retention. Maintain catheter. PSA, repeat creatinine levels. Urinalysis. Renal and pelvic ultrasound.

Note 44

Progress note day 2

CC: Asthma

Patient reports improved breathing overnight. No additional attacks. Slept well. On exam, appears in no acute distress, wheezes are decreased. RRR. Scheduled bronchial challenge test for today. Spirometry results were worse than testing 6 months ago. D/C magnesium sulfate.

Note 45

IP D2

Patient reports pelvic pain has resolved. Good urine output from Foley. Renal U/S negative. Pelvic U/S image shows significant increase in BPH. Recommend TURP. Reviewed with patient and wife, scheduled for tomorrow.

Note 46

Hospital day 10

CC: Pain

Patient reports increased swelling and constant pain in abdomen due to ascites. Pain is reduced when the patient lies on her side. Sleep is interrupted and not restful. Patient reports feeling depressed and hopeless due to her worsening cirrhosis.
Patient is tearful, in moderate distress. Shallow, rapid breathing. Abdomen is grossly swollen, positive wave, bulging flanks, shifting dullness.
Grade 3 ascites secondary to alcoholic cirrhosis. Resident will complete paracentesis later today. Albumin IV. Will discuss TIPS again with the patient to see if she is amenable to the procedure.

Note 47

Progress day 2

CC: Suppressed appetite

Patient continues to have little interested in food. She says many of the foods offered nauseate her. The foods that are palatable, she only wants to eat a few bites of before reporting satiety. Patient denies depression, feelings of hopelessness, chest pain, shortness of breath, dizziness, musculoskeletal pain. On exam, VSS, patient appears thin, gaunt. Patient's mood is significantly depressed, but she refuses any medication due to denial of diagnosis. Elderly failure to thrive. Continue to encourage caloric goal and variety of food offerings. Waiting for POA to arrive from out of town to discuss possibility of medication, g-tube.

Note 48

Dear Dr. Smith,

Thank you for asking me to see your patient regarding possible hypothyroidism. I saw her today in clinic. She is a pleasant 52-year-old woman with primary complaint of fatigue ×6 months. She is so fatigued that she regularly requires an afternoon nap. She also reports often feeling cold and recent 20 lb weight gain. She has increased her exercise to walking 20 minutes 5 days a week without any improvement in her fatigue. If anything, she feels more fatigue after walking. No history of radiation treatments. She has a sister with hypothyroidism. No tobacco/moderate ETOH.

On exam, patient is overweight, HEENT normal. Thyroid is slightly enlarged. Trachea midline. Skin pale and dry. Mild weakness in grip strength. Brittle nails. AAO × 3.

Hypothyroidism evident in labs.

Hypothyroidism. Patient will begin Levothyroxine treatment and see me in a month.

Sincerely,

Dr. Jones

Note 49

Requesting physician: Dr. Smith
Reason for consultation: atypical chest wall pain

History

Patient has a 6-month history of chest pain that occurs randomly without any identified precursor. Pain feels centered more in the chest wall than within the chest. Pain usually starts on the flank and radiates, encompassing the entire chest and sometimes the thoracic back. It may begin on one or both sides, and lasts up to 10 minutes before spontaneously resolving. The pain is bad enough that the patient must stop moving and talking until it resolved. Patient has tried to resolve with tums and chewable aspirin with no effect. Patient sometimes is also diaphoretic. No nausea, no vomiting. No dizziness. No typical chest pain or shortness of breath. No GU symptoms. Positive for fibromyalgia which results in disturbed sleep patterns, joint pain, fatigue. Patient reports anxiety controlled with medication. Cannot recall if pain results from increased stress. No polyuria, no polydipsia.

Med list

Citalopram 20 mg qd
Melatonin 3 mg an hour before bedtime
Cetirizine 10 mg qd
Benadryl as needed for allergic symptoms
800 mg ibuprofen tid for chronic pain
No tobacco/social ETOH
No family history of heart disease or stroke

Exam

NAD, VSS. HEENT normal. RRR. Lungs CTAB. Unable to reproduce the pain by palpating the chest wall. GI normal. Neuro normal. AAO×3, mood is anxious. No enlarged cervical or axillary lymph nodes.

Pain is likely secondary to fibromyalgia. Discussed adding Cymbalta to patient's medication regime, which she found reasonable. Will begin therapy and return in 1 month. Patient agreed to keep a pain journal until the next appointment so we can identify any patterns.

Cc: Dr. Smith

Note 50

PCP: Dr. Smith

CC: Oral lesions

Patient is seen for the first time in the ID clinic today. New complaint of oral lesions with underlying HIV status. Patient reports considerable pain at the lesion sites when eating spicy food. Also reports altered taste of foods. Patient has tried to resolve the lesions by avoiding troublesome foods and regular mouthwash use. Patient reports some recent weight loss due to lack of appetite. Occasional night sweats. Patient reports a residual cough from URI.

Denies any symptoms in eyes, card, GI, GU, neuro, psych, ms, skin.

Patient reports good compliance with medications. HIV status for 8 years. No family history of oral cancers. No tobacco/no ETOH.

Patient is NAD. Head normocephalic, atraumatic. Eyes, ears, nose, facial skin normal. Enlarged cervical nodes. Mouth shows flat red patches on palate and dorsal tongue. Vestibule clear. Good dentition with some gingivitis. No upper body lesions. RRR. Lungs slight ronchi bilaterally. AAOx3. Neuro grossly normal.

Assessment and plan

1. HIV Stage II. Labs drawn today. T-cells likely falling.
2. Erythematous candidiasis vs. KS vs. erythoplakia, likely candidiasis. Samples sent to pathology. Prescribed clotrimazole topical as a precaution. Will adjust treatment based on pathology results.
3. Cough. Ordered chest x-ray.

Will see the patient back in 1 week, or as soon as the pathology results are available.

CC: Dr. Smith

Note 51

AID Consult

[Note documented in shared record]

Attending service requested we see their patient for persistent hives at the IV site. Patient reports rash has been intermittently present over the past 4 days. It seems to occur after a specific drug is administered. When it occurs, the rash is itchy. Patient does not report difficulty breathing, dizziness or lightheadedness, increased heart rate, swelling in the mouth or throat, nausea, vomiting, or abdominal pain. No environmental allergies.

On exam, VSS. HEENT normal. IV site is red, maybe some residual hives.

A/P: Mild drug allergy. Continue course ordered by attending.

Note 52

GI Consult

[Note documented in shared record]

Attending service noted an incidental finding of stomach mass. Saw the patient today, a pleasant 12-year-old girl. She reports some occasional stomach upset. Mom reports what is likely indigestion. Mom notes that the patient often chews her hair or sucks on a lock of hair. On exam patient's abdomen is normal. Review of the x-ray image shows probable trichobezoar. Will schedule the patient for endoscopic removal tomorrow.

Note 53

Patient presented to the ED with a swollen lt knee ×10 days. It is worse at the end of the day. Patient has attempted RICE with minimal effect. Does not recall an initiating event. Contralateral knee is unaffected. No numbness, no tingling. Foot does not feel cold. Able to bear some weight without pain. No recent weight change. No cardiovascular personal or family history.

Exam
VSS. Knee is stable, swollen, no redness, dry, not hot, unable to reproduce any pain on palpation. Full ROM lt hip, no pain. Lt ankle normal. Normal pedal pulses. Contralateral leg unaffected.

Assessment and plan
Knee pain with unknown etiology. Supplied sleeve. Provided work leave note and referral to orthopod. Continue RICE, following it closely. Minimal walking.

Note 54

Patient presented to the ED with 2-day complaint of increasing sharp LLQ pain and associated frequent gas. Reports a fever, decreased appetite, and mild nausea. No vomiting, no chills, no chest pain, no sob. Last bowel movement was yesterday. No personal history of IBD.
Patient appears in moderate distress, slightly diaphoretic. Heart rate is regular, increased pulse. Lungs normal. Significant pain on palpation in LLQ. Other three quadrants normal, no organomegaly, positive bowel sounds. External genitalia appear normal. No hernias. AAO × 3.

Labs
Increased white count

CT report
Sigmoid colon shows localized thickening and hyperemia, inflammatory changes. Noted diverticulae.

Assessment and plan
Diverticulitis. Discussed patient with GI attending and agreed patient should be admitted to their service.

Note 55

Patient presents to ED with complaint of painful toe ×2 weeks that has been increasing. Patient describes the pain as feeling like someone is trying to peel his toenail off. No numbness, no tingling. Patient is not diabetic.

Right greater toenail has a foul odor, is discolored, thickened, and crumbly. Other nails are unaffected. Patient has a fungal infection in the toe. Prescribed Lamisil for the infection and recommended ibuprofen for pain. Encourage the patient to select a primary care physician and follow-up with their office rather than the ED.

Note 56

I saw the patient for the first time today in his assisted living apartment. Patient has had increasing right hip/leg pain over the past year. Patient did not suffer a fall or other trauma that precipitated the pain. Pain increases when the patient stands for a length of time or tries to walk further than 100 feet. No change in bowel or bladder. No fever, no change in appetite. Patient lives with his wife of 48 years.

Note 56—cont'd

On exam, VSS, RRR, CTAB, positive pedal pulses. Bilat knees and ankles normal. Hips, good ROM. Unable to isolate pain while patient is sitting. Positive pain when patient sits on bed with legs straight out and lifts affected leg. Upon standing and having the patient walk, he is able to describe and isolate the location of the pain. Reduced reflexes in affected leg.

Patient likely has sciatica due to spinal stenosis. I've ask him to go for an x-ray to confirm. Instructed patient in using ice, heat, and ibuprofen. Will have activity coordinator stop by to show the patient some exercises to strengthen his core muscles, which should also help. Patient is encouraged not to rest in bed and to stay active.

Note 57

I saw the patient again today in the assisted living facility. Today, she has a complaint of a lump under the skin of her thigh. She noticed it a couple of months ago. It has increased slightly over time. She is able to move it freely under the skin. It is not in itself painful, but it can press on something else in her arm that causes mild pain. She doesn't see any redness. It doesn't feel hot. It doesn't cause any numbness or tingling. She has never noticed a lump like this before.

On exam, the mass moves freely under the skin, measures about 1.5 cm diameter. I am not able to re-produce an pain with palpation. No other masses were noted on the thighs, bilateral forearms, or trunk. Blood pressure was slightly elevated today.

I reassured the patient that this mass is a lipoma, or fatty tumor. It does not need treatment at this time. I encouraged her to let me know if it continues to grow, becomes painful, or restricts movement. If it is cosmetically unappealing, she can consider removal.

Note 58

This is a new patient to our house calls practice. Patient complains of hearing a high-pitched "tinging" noise without any external source. The sound has been presents for many years, but has been more troublesome over the past year. Patient describes the noise as similar to the noise an old tube television made. Patient is not able to make the sound better or worse. It does not interfere with the patient's ability to hear normally, except the patient may have some trouble hearing a conversation in a crowd. No other ear complaints. No eye complaints. No nose, mouth, or throat complaints.

Patient's head is normocephalic, atraumatic. Eyes normal. Nose and mouth normal. Ears, appear nor-mal externally. No middle ear obstructions. No sign of infection, no redness. Tympanic membranes are clear bilaterally. Patient can hear tuning fork bilaterally.

Tinnitus—Described the condition to the patient and some potential relief through use of white noise and cognitive behavioral therapy. Patient asked about taking a lipoflavinoid supplement, which I noted has not been found to definitively treat tinnitus, but would not adversely affect the patient. I will refer the patient for CBT on request.

Note 59

This new patient to our practice was seen today at home. She is concerned about a lesion on her cheek. It's been growing, first appearing about 6 months ago. She hasn't noticed any other lesions. The lesion is about 8mm in diameter at its widest, but is asymmetrical. The borders are irregular and color is blue and black. Highly suspicious for melanoma. I've asked the patient to come in for a biopsy tomorrow.

Note 60

Saw the patient in follow-up today at home. Patient has been struggling with hemorrhoids. They are itchy and occasionally bleed. The patient has been attempting a variety of home treatments including sitz baths and OTC cream, which have provided some relief but has not eliminated symptoms.

The patient's symptoms are significant enough that I would like to treat the hemorrhoids with banding, but the patient has declined. Will continue with home treatments and monitor. I have encouraged the patient to contact me if bleeding or pain increase and that we can treat them anytime he would like.

Note 61

Saw the patient at home in follow-up today for her pseudovertigo. Patient reports considerable improvement after taking citalopram for a month. Her symptoms are occurring less often. Her vital signs are stable today. Eyes are clear, no nystagmus. AAO×3 with some mild anxiety. Patient feels her symptoms are adequately controlled. Will continue citalopram 20 mg pd. Have discussed slightly increasing her dosage if she finds symptoms are not controlled.

Note 62

78-year-old patient presents to ED with 5-day history of fever, ache, increasing cough and nasal congestion. Patient also notes extreme fatigue feeling "like I was hit by a bus". Eyes have been watery, positive for headache. Patient did not get a flu shot this season.

Increased heart rate. Patient appears flushed and slightly diaphoretic. Eyes are injected. Ears, nose, mouth, normal. Bilateral wheezes, normal respiration rate, no retractions. Patient reports achiness when joints are manipulated. AAO×3. Neuro grossly normal. Abdomen is soft, non-tender, positive bowel sounds, no organomegaly.

Patient has presumed influenza. Admit for aggressive treatment given the advanced state of symptoms.

Note 63

3-year-old patient presents with his mother to the ED this evening. Mother noticed the patient sniffling constantly for about two hours. Suspects the patient may have put a bead up his nose. No eye symptoms, no cough, no fever.

On exam, the patient is pleasant and cooperative, alert and responsive. Nasal inspection reveals a bead lodged in the left nare.

The bead was removed with forceps. Patient was encouraged to not put anything in the nose in the future.

Note 64

Existing patient in the practice presents with his mother with 3-day history of itchy, red eye. Patient has crusty eyes in the morning. Mother thinks he was exposed to viral conjunctivitis at school.

Eyes are obviously reddened. ENMT normal. No cervical nodes.

Presumed viral conjunctivitis. Patient should remain at home until symptoms clear. Prescribed an antibacterial drop as a precautionary measure. Launder pillow cases. Do not touch eyes. Good hand washing.

Note 65

Patient presents to the clinic today for follow-up of her Guillain-Barre syndrome. Patient has been working through recovery for about 6 months now. She continues to feel improved. Primary symptoms include limb weakness, low blood pressure, and blurred vision. AON. History includes concurrent mononucleosis. No tobacco/no ETOH.

Patient presents today in no acute distress. HEENT is normal except for mild vision blurring. RRR, CTAB. Strength is still weak in all four limbs, but improved from last visit. Reflexes are depressed x4 limbs, no numbness, no tingling. AAO×3. No lymphadenopathy.

Patient's recovery is continuing to improve. Patient will continue physical therapy and see us back in 2 months.

Note 66

Patient is new to the dermatology clinic today. Patient is concerned about red, itchy skin on her left ante-cubital fossa following use of an adhesive bandage for 1 day following blood donation. Patient has noticed increased sensitivity to adhesives in the past year or so. No fever, no chills. No other skin sensitivities. No recent cold symptoms. Patient does not have environmental allergies.

On exam, VSS. Skin on arm is still reddened and inflamed at site of adhesive bandage. No other skin irritations present.

Patient has a generalized skin sensitivity to adhesives. Should avoid adhesive bandages in the future and if they are necessary, use them as little as possible. Patient should wash the affected area with warm soapy water, ensuring removal of all adhesive material. Prescribed steroid cream. Emphasized using the cream according to directions to prevent further skin irritation.

Note 67

New patient presents to the office today complaining of a persistent dark spot in the vision of her left eye for 1 month. The spot appeared spontaneously. No associated pain. No trauma to the eye. The patient describes the spot as like a sperm, with a head and a squiggly tail. When she tries to look at it, the spot moves and she is unable to look directly at the spot. No history of similar spots or of other eye disease.

On exam with slit lamp, the affected eye has a vitriolic floater. The contralateral eye is unaffected.

Assured the patient that vitriolic floaters are common with age, as the solid parts of the vitreous will occasionally congeal. The spot will probably dissipate over the next few months, but may not disappear completely. Recommended the patient make an appointment for a full eye exam.

Note 68

Patients presents to the clinic today with concerns regarding persistent anxiety. The patient reports constant worry that affects her ability to get to sleep at night. She feels she becomes too concerned about stressors and "can't let go" of things at what she feels is an appropriate level. Her husband tells her it has been worse over the past year. Sometimes she worries so much that she experiences heart palpitations and stomachache. Patient has no history of diagnosed anxiety or depression. Patient does not report suicidal ideation. No tobacco/3-4 drinks per week. Does not drink to excess when anxiety is high.

On exam, patient is pleasant and in no acute distress, VSS but bp is elevated. Rechecked bp at the end of the visit and it was normal. On questioning, I confirmed absence of suicidal ideation. Patient has social anxieties about crowds and describes some obsessive-compulsive disorder behaviors. Nails are bitten down, but not inflamed. Patient's main concerns center around her work.

The patient has generalized anxiety disorder. The patient was interested in trying a medication along with talk therapy. I prescribed citalopram 20mg today along with a referral to a therapist. She will follow-up with me in 1 month.

■ **ADVANCED**

Notes in this section may not be billable. If not, note why. There may be other unusual situations or coding methods necessary in this section.

Note 69

New patient presents to the clinic today concerned with possible high blood pressure. His father had high blood pressure and died of a stroke at 68 years old. The patient has had some elevated blood pressure readings in the past. He just turned 40 and decided it would be good to check on this. The patient completed a health assessment form, which we reviewed together. *[Form is in the record and includes a comprehensive ROS and PFSH.]*

On exam, patient's initial and repeat blood pressure readings were elevated. Heart RRR. Lungs CTAB. Moderate JVD.

We had a long discussion regarding high blood pressure and its effects. With the history of elevated readings and today's readings, I want to first try to moderate his readings with diet and exercise. We discussed eliminating excess sodium from his diet, with an emphasis on avoiding processed foods. I'd like to see him do some aerobic exercise for at least 30 minutes a day 5 days a week. Patient will also purchase a home blood pressure monitor and keep a journal of readings. I'll see him back in a month.

Note 70

Patient admitted to obs to monitor CHF. Patient has a 2-day hx of SOB and CP due to CHF. This is the worst his symptoms have ever been. Patient takes Lasix, Prilosec, and naproxen sodium.

On exam, patient's breathing is labored, crackles present bil. Heart rate is irregular. Positive edema bil lower legs. Positive pedal pulses bil, but decreased.

EKG is abnormal. Labs are elevated. Abd CT ordered. Heart cath scheduled for tomorrow.

CHF. Monitor overnight. Continue meds.

Note 71

Hospital day 7

CC: Asthma

Patient continues to improve. Patient reports minimal wheezing with respiration and is able to walk around the unit with ease. Sleeping well. Good appetite. VSS. O2 Sats 99% on room air. Resp CTAB except very minor wheezing. Will discharge this afternoon with instructions for follow-up.

Note 72

The patient presents at the clinic for follow-up of uncontrolled DM II. We spent the entire visit discussing the importance of compliance with the treatment plan and barriers to compliance including pain with sticks, food preferences, and eating out. Our total time together today was 20 minutes.

Note 73

Patient presents with intractable vomiting x18 hours. Patient vomits about every 30 minutes. The patient is not able to even keep sips of water down. No chest pain, no shortness of breath, no fever, positive diaphoresis, no diarrhea, no blood in urine. No history of peptic ulcer.

VSS, no GI tenderness. Treated with Phenergan and Zofran with relief. Instructions for hydration and BRAT diet. ED discharge 2238.

Note 74

Dr. Jones asked me to see this patient regarding pediatric asthma. Patient has had asthma symptoms for 3 years. Patient notices symptoms worsen in cold air and with exertion.
On exam, patient has remote wheezes bilaterally. No retractions.
Patient has typical asthmatic symptoms. Seems well controlled on current meds, no changes. Nothing more I can offer.
cc: Dr. Jones

Note 75

Well-known patient presents to clinic today with right lower quadrant pain that started last night, starting near her navel and then moving towards the right lower quadrant. She reports the pain as 8/10. Also reports subjective fever. Normal bowel movements. No unusual food yesterday, all homemade. Pain is worse with movement. No musculoskeletal pain. Normal urine output, no blood in urine. Last menstrual period 10 days ago.

Exam: Patient is in obvious distress, doubled over guarding the lower abdomen. VSS with low-grade fever of 100.7 elevated pulse. Eyes clear. Mucous membranes moist and pink. RRR. Lungs CTAB. Abdomen is soft, no scars, no lesions, no rashes, bowel sounds are present in all four quadrants. Extremely tender to palpation across lower abdomen, less so in upper abdomen. Tympanic in three quadrants. Patient could not tolerate RLQ percussion. No organomegaly. Moderate lower abdomen rebound tenderness. No CVA tenderness. Psoas sign was very positive for abdominal pain. Positive obturator sign.

Patient has presumed acute appendicitis vs ovarian cyst. Negative urine pregnancy test in office. Called the hospital and will send her over via private car for direct admit. Ordered labs and CT upon arrival.

[Later the same day, the same physician sees the patient in the hospital. This is the inpatient note from the hospital medical record.]

Patient continues to have significant guarding. Stable RLQ pain is 8/10. No nausea/vomiting/diarrhea.

Labs and CT consistent with acute appendicitis. Surgery has been consulted, transfer of care to surgery service.

Note 76

[This note is documented in a shared electronic medical record.]
Consult request by nephrology attending Dr. Smith to assess oral ulcerations.

CC: Oral ulcerations

The patient is a pleasant 53-year-old diabetic with episodic oral ulcerations. She has been experiencing them for approximately 2 years. They cause her significant pain when eating. Patient has had some recent weight loss due to a lack of appetite during ulcer outbreaks. No joint pain, no skin ulcerations, no difficulty swallowing. I reviewed the Dr. Smith's admission PFSH with the patient and it is unchanged today.

Continued

Note 76—cont'd

On exam the patient is a patient black female in no apparent distress. Her head is normocephalic. Eyes are clear. Mucous membranes are pink and moist. Three red, craterized ulcerations noted in the oral vestibule. Two ulcers noted on tongue. Consistent with diabetic oral ulcers. Heart is normal. Breath sounds are equal. No skin ulcerations noted.

Apthous ulcers. Wrote orders for Peroxyl and benzocaine. Discussed with the patient the importance of good oral hygiene and use of treatments after discharge. Patient will follow-up with me in clinic prn.

Note 77

Postop day 1. Patient reports moderate pain, well-controlled with PCA morphine. Incision sites healing well. Continue to monitor fracture sites, wean PCA.

Note 78

Patient was admitted to obs this morning with left lower leg cellulitis. Patient scraped his leg on a rock while swimming in a lake. Admitted for IV treatment and monitoring injury for aggressive infection. Treatment was completed and successful. Patient was discharged home in the evening with instructions to monitor the wound.

Note 79

Inpatient Day 12

Patient has no complaints overnight. Appetite is better.
VSS

Gen: morbidly obese, resting in bed in NAD

CV: RRR, no m/g/r, 2+ pulses

Pulm: CTAB

Skin: large area of denuded skin right lower leg, yellowish drainage, edema improving

A&P Morbid obesity with cellulitis of RLE

Note 80

Nursing Facility Admission

87-year-old patient admitted to the Alzheimer's unit today. According to the patient's daughter, he was diagnosed over 15 years ago. Disease has progressed to the point where the patient is unable to care for himself and his daughter is also no longer to care for him properly. She fears he will fall and she won't be able to help him. Patient is largely averbal and all available history is given by his daughter. Health assessment form was completed by his daughter, which we discussed. *[Form is on the record and includes 14 system review and complete PFSH.]*

Note 80—cont'd

On exam, the patient is a pleasant, thin man in no apparent distress. He is not oriented. He answers some questions with a nod or an incorrect mumbled comment. RRR, CTAB. Posture is stooped. Weak grip strength bilateral. Positive pedal pulses. Reduced LE reflexes. No rashes no lesions no skin breaks. No lymphadenopathy.

Patient has stage 7 Alzheimer's disease. Patient is very healthy otherwise with no medications. Patient needs support of daily living tasks and monitoring. Ordered OT.

Note 81

ED note ankle template

Patient presents with left ankle pain so bad she cannot bear weight on the leg. She came in immediately following stepping on the edge of a sidewalk and falling, inverting the ankle. No knee pain, no shoulder pain, no other complaints. No numbness, no tingling. NKDA. On exam, the ankle is red, swollen, and tight. Considerable pain on attempt to move the ankle.

X-ray doesn't show any fracture. Splinted the ankle and referred patient to an orthopod in 3 days.

Note 82

CC: Concussion

HPI

30-year-old female restrained passenger in a two-vehicle collision presented to the emergency department via local fire department rescue squad from crash site at 5:10p.m. Upon arrival she was combative but coherent, complaining of 9/10 pain on the right side of her head. She reports hitting the side of her head against the passenger side window during impact. She has generalized achiness, but no other reported injuries or symptoms. She was admitted to observation last night to continue monitoring effects of the concussion. Today, she remains in observation status. Since last night, the patient is more alert. Continues to report right-sided head pain, as well as right shoulder soreness and generalized achiness. History was collected from the patient and her significant other.

ROS

Eyes: difficulty focusing

Card: no chest pain

Resp: no breathing difficulties

GI: two episodes of vomiting overnight, none for about three hours

GU: no hematuria. Voiding well.

Neuro: struggles to concentrate on one thought for too long. No seizure activity.

Psych: no abnormal thought, no hallucinations

Exam

Eyes: considerable nystagmus, pupils equal, round, and reactive to light

ENMT: mucous membranes moist

Card: RRR

Resp: CTAB

Continued

Note 82—cont'd

GI: non-tender, no guarding, no rebound

Musculo: weak tone, as expected

Psych: AAO×3

Neuro: cranial nerves intact, no sign of seizure activity

A/P:
Order updated labs, PT assessment, OT assessment, repeat CT.
Continue to monitor ongoing concussion symptoms. If sleeping, arouse hourly. Monitor I/O. Will determine tomorrow a.m. whether to admit or discharge.

Note 83

Patient presents with complaint of multiple insect bites on legs. They occurred about an hour ago. Patient is worried they are poisonous bites or that she is having an allergic reaction. No known history of insect bite allergy. Bites look red, but are typical of mosquito bites. Encouraged the patient to wear long pants in the evenings and to apply calamine lotion and use oral Benadryl to reduce symptoms.

Note 84

Asked to see the patient by her pediatrician here in the genetics clinic. Patient is a 3-year-old bubbly girl here with her parents for results of genetic testing. Results showed the patient does have genetic markers of achondrodysplasia. I discussed at length with her parents some of the complications of the condition including hydrocephalus, spinal stenosis, and short stature. Her father also has achondrodysplasia and is familiar with various treatments and challenges of the disease. The family was positive about the patient's prognosis and fully prepared to support her as she grows. It was a pleasure to meet with this family. We spent a total of 35 minutes together today. *[Documented in shared record.]*

Note 85

Good Samaritan Nursing Home

Patient is 88-year-old male resident with new CVA ×7 days. Experiencing right hemiplegia and aphasia, therefore unable to complete history with patient. Nurses state he has been resting comfortably with little agitation.

VSS. Weight unchanged from last visit. Patient seems aware of the visit and attempts to answer yes/no questions with head nods and other gestures. Eyes unremarkable. Mucous membranes moist. RRR. Lungs CTAB. Abd soft non-tender positive bowel sounds. Right-sided weakness unable to wiggle toes. Left-side limited range of motion but adequate sensation.

Completed updated MDS/RAI. New CVA with right hemiplegia and aphasia. PT/OT orders written. Ordered follow-up labs. Discussed the patient's prognosis with the patient's neurologist.

Note 86

History: patient presents today to establish care with our practice. 49-year-old female without major complaint. See patient health assessment form for complete ROS and PFSH reviewed with patient *[Form is included in record.]*

Exam: VSS, patient is a 49-year-old lean female in no acute distress

HEENT: normal

Neck: no lymphadenopathy, trachea midline, thyroid normal

Card: RRR, no m/g/r

Resp: CTAB

Breast: normal

GI: no tenderness, no guarding, no rebound, positive bowel sounds in all quadrants, no organomegaly

GU: deferred

Neurological: grossly normal

Psychological: Alert and oriented × 3

Skin: no unusual lesions or rashes

Risk assessment: Patient wears her seatbelt 100%
Ordered fasting lipids. Nurse will administer pertussis adult booster and tetanus.
Discussed with patient importance of maintaining an active lifestyle, regular mammogram screenings, onset of menopause. Patient will return in the fall for an influenza vaccine and schedule a 1-year follow-up.

Note 87

New patient in the office today complains of bilateral foot pain. Pain has been present for a couple of years, slowly increasing. The pain has been bad enough in the past couple of months that the patient is purchasing wider shoes and avoiding certain shoes. No history of foot surgery or foot fracture. Mother suffered from bilateral bunions. On exam the patient is suffering bilateral hallux valgus. The patient's condition is severe enough that surgical correction is recommended. Will schedule as soon as the patient can arrange time off from work.

Note 88

Patient was admitted to our service today with late stage AIDS. Patient's primary concern today is failure to thrive. Patient has no appetite and has been losing weight and strength for a couple of months. Patient's caregivers have tried supplementing the patient's calories with Ensure, but patient is just not interested in eating. When patient has a bowel movement it is diarrheal. Patient usually feels very cold and finds it difficult to get warm. NKDA. No tobacco/no ETOH/no illicits.

Blood pressure is low. Heart rate is elevated. Respirations are slow. Patient appears gaunt but in no apparent distress. Skin is papery. No hair loss. No mouth lesions. Eyes clear. Muscles show wasting. Patient has widespread lymphadenopathy. Lungs are rather clear, but patient has a persistent cough. Liver is enlarged. No GI pain on palpation. Patient is AAO×3 but significantly depressed.

Will try to keep the patient hydrated and work with the patient to determine whether we should attempt to improve patient's caloric intake or if he wants to withdraw care.

Note 89

Our diabetic nurse went to see the patient in his assisted living apartment today. The patient has a new diagnosis of DM II 2 weeks ago. The patient isn't experiencing any sides effects. He reports a moderate diet, but could cut his carbs. No visual changes. The nurse reports his vital signs were stable. The nurse had a long discussion with the patient regarding blood checks, diet, exercise, foot care, and regular medical check-ups.

Note 90

Code from memory a recent visit by you or a family member to a physician office. Consider each component of an E&M service, what you were asked, what the physician examined, what the physician ordered or prescribed, the diagnosis. Should the visit have been billed based on time rather than key components?

Note 91

Patient presents to the office today for the first time complaining of snoring. His wife states he snores loud enough that it will wake her up. The snoring has been worse since he gained weight in the last 6 months or so. His wife is worried that his breathing pauses during his snoring. He was also told years ago that he has deviated septum. Will schedule the patient for a sleep study in our lab.

Note 92

Inpatient day 10

Primary concern today is the patient's continuing fever. History is unchanged from yesterday's note. *[Yesterday's note includes a detailed history.]* Temp is still elevated. RRR. Lungs clear. Fever is not improving. Ordering additional labs.

Note 93

Patient just moved to the area and comes in to the office today for the first time. She suffers from environmental allergies and needs a new prescription for her medication. The patient was tested for allergies when she was younger and found to have a number of environmental sensitivities. She is able to maintain good control with Clarinex. She doesn't like to use eye drops or nasal sprays. No runny nose or itchy eyes today. On exam, nares are clear, ears are clear. Recommended that the patient may have different allergies in this area and would benefit from new allergy testing. Gave her a referral for an allergist and a refill script.

Note 94

Patient arrived in the ED unresponsive immediately following a tackle during a football game. The patient was hit and fell to the ground. He was rousable but not alert on site. GCS 5, extension to painful stimuli, incomprehensible sounds. Neck is immobilized. Unable to obtain additional history due to patient condition. Head is normocephalic, atraumatic. No facial abrasions. Nose is symmetrical. No rhinorrhea, no rhinohemorrhagia, no otorrhea, no blood in mouth. Dentition intact. Unable to examine neck due to c-collar. Full ROM arms, legs. Chest on x-ray no rib fractures. Abdomen is soft. Weak rectal tone. Patient appears to have lost bladder control. We spent 45 minutes stabilizing the patient including constant attention in CT to be ready to attend any sudden decompensation. Patient remained unresponsive throughout. Transferred the patient to the trauma team for admission.

Note 95

Visited the patient today in his assisted living apartment to discuss his weakness. Patient reports weakness is about the same as last time. He tries to do his exercises every day. His grip strength was about the same as last time. We spent a majority of the 40 minute visit discussing the patient's interest in improving his strength, strategies for that, whether his living arrangement was providing him appropriate support. I'll see him again in a month.

Note 96

Palliative care service was asked to see the inpatient today regarding end of life care. We spent 35 minutes talking.

Note 97

Day 3: 7:30 a.m.
Patient received a 3rd-degree burn on his right arm following a kitchen grease incident. Today, the patient's main complaint is pain in the arm since yesterday. He feels the morphine is wearing off before he is able to use the PCA again. Agreed that the PCA is set at too long of an interval. Ordered the PCA reset. Will see the patient this afternoon to see if the pain is improved.
Day 3: 4:15pm
Saw the patient again this afternoon to check on his pain control. Patient says the control is much better. He is not feeling over sedated. On exam, the burn wound is looking as expected. Vital signs are stable, no signs of infection. Will take the patient to OR for sedated dressing changes in the morning.

Note 98

[Note is entered in a shared medical record of a multi-specialty practice.]

ENT clinic note

Patient is a 3-year-old charming boy that Dr. Kim asked me to see regarding treatment for otitis media. No current ear pain. Tympanic membrane shows evidence of chronic inflammation. Patient has chronic otitis media. Will schedule patient for tympanostomy.

Note 99

Patient returns today after 10 day antibiotic treatment for tonsillitis. Patient reports symptoms have resolved. On exam throat is normal. Patient will gargle regularly with salt water and use good hand hygiene.

Note 100

New patient comes in to the office today with upper body comedopapular acne ×3 years. Facial skin shows a diffuse profusion of comedopapular acne, which extends down the neck, across the chest to approximately the nipple line, and down the thoracic back. Some areas show early scarring, especially where the patient notes repeated disturbance of lesions by scratching and expression. Patient notes these lesions are often itchy and difficult not to scratch. The acne does not extend down the arms or otherwise on the body. On the upper back, larger lesions are painful when the surrounding skin is palpated. Patient denies that the acne is associated with any joint pain or achiness. Mucous membranes pink and moist. Over-the-counter medications have not been effective. NKDA. Will begin Accutane regimen.

Note 101

Patient is a 74-year-old male admitted today with pneumonia. Symptoms began about 10 days ago including productive cough, fever, fatigue, and chills. The patient reports symptoms as 7/10. Patient tried a number of over-the-counter medications before seeking treatment.

Const: fever. Oxygen sats 92% on room air. 100% on nasal cannula.
Cervical lymph nodes mildly swollen.

Resp: inspirations show mild distress. On percussion, chest is dull. Decreased air intake. Mild wheezes. No rales. Rust colored sputum.

Assessment and plan: chest x-ray positive for pneumonia. Likely bacterial pneumonia, but have sent sputum to lab to see if anything grows out. Antibiotics ordered.

Note 102

Patient returns to the clinic today following 1 month of treatment for GI reflux. Patient reports symptoms are much improved. The patient notices a difference if he forgets to take his medication. We reviewed a list of foods to avoid, as well as trying to lose some weight, which would improve his symptoms. Continue with Nexium. I'll see him back in 6 months.

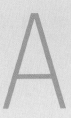

1995 Documentation Guidelines for Evaluation and Management Services*

◼ I. WHAT IS DOCUMENTATION AND WHY IS IT IMPORTANT?

Medical record documentation is required to record pertinent facts, findings, and observations about an individual's health history including past and present illnesses, examinations, tests, treatments, and outcomes. The medical record chronologically documents the care of the patient and is an important element contributing to high quality care. The medical record facilitates:

- the ability of the physician and other health care professionals to evaluate and plan the patient's immediate treatment, and to monitor his/her health care over time;
- communication and continuity of care among physicians and other health care professionals involved in the patient's care;
- accurate and timely claims review and payment;
- appropriate utilization review and quality of care evaluations; and
- collection of data that may be useful for research and education.

An appropriately documented medical record can reduce many of the "hassles" associated with claims processing and may serve as a legal document to verify the care provided, if necessary.

◼ WHAT DO PAYERS WANT AND WHY?

Because payers have a contractual obligation to enrollees, they may require reasonable documentation that services are consistent with the insurance coverage provided. They may request information to validate:

- the site of service;
- the medical necessity and appropriateness of the diagnostic and/or therapeutic services provided;
- and/or that services provided have been accurately reported.

---

*Adapted from 1995 Documentation Guidelines For Evaluation and Management Services, Centers for Medicare & Medicaid Services, www.cms.gov/ (search "1995 documentation guidelines")

▪ II. GENERAL PRINCIPLES OF MEDICAL RECORD DOCUMENTATION

The principles of documentation listed below are applicable to all types of medical and surgical services in all settings. For Evaluation and Management (E/M) services, the nature and amount of physician work and documentation varies by type of service, place of service and the patient's status. The general principles listed below may be modified to account for these variable circumstances in providing E/M services.

1. The medical record should be complete and legible.

2. The documentation of each patient encounter should include:

- reason for the encounter and relevant history, physical examination findings, and prior diagnostic test results;
- assessment, clinical impression, or diagnosis;
- plan for care; and
- date and legible identity of the observer.

3. If not documented, the rationale for ordering diagnostic and other ancillary services should be easily inferred.

4. Past and present diagnoses should be accessible to the treating and/or consulting physician.

5. Appropriate health risk factors should be identified.

6. The patient's progress, response to and changes in treatment, and revision of diagnosis should be documented.

7. The CPT and ICD-9-CM codes reported on the health insurance claim form or billing statement should be supported by the documentation in the medical record.

▪ III. DOCUMENTATION OF E/M SERVICES

This publication provides definitions and documentation guidelines for the three *key* components of E/M services and for visits which consist predominately of counseling or coordination of care. The three key components—history, examination, and medical decision making—appear in the descriptors for office and other outpatient services, hospital observation services, hospital inpatient services, consultations, emergency department services, nursing facility services, domiciliary care services, and home services. While some of the text of CPT has been repeated in this publication, the reader should refer to CPT for the complete descriptors for E/M services and instructions for selecting a level of service. **Documentation guidelines are identified by bold-italic *DG*.**

The descriptors for the levels of E/M services recognize seven components which are used in defining the levels of E/M services. These components are:

- history;
- examination;
- medical decision making;
- counseling;
- coordination of care;
- nature of presenting problem; and
- time.

The first three of these components (i.e., history, examination and medical decision making) are the *key* components in selecting the level of E/M services. An exception to this rule is the case of visits which consist predominantly of counseling or coordination of care; for these services time is the key or controlling factor to qualify for a particular level of E/M service.

For certain groups of patients, the recorded information may vary slightly from that described here. Specifically, the medical records of infants, children, adolescents and pregnant women may have additional or modified information recorded in each history and examination area.

As an example, newborn records may include under history of the present illness (HPI) the details of mother's pregnancy and the infant's status at birth; social history will focus on family structure; family history will focus on congenital anomalies and hereditary disorders in the family. In addition, information on growth and development and/or nutrition will be recorded. Although not specifically defined in these documentation guidelines, these patient group variations on history and examination are appropriate.

A. Documentation of History

The levels of E/M services are based on four types of history (Problem Focused, Expanded Problem Focused, Detailed, and Comprehensive). Each type of history includes some or all of the following elements:

- Chief complaint (CC);

- History of present illness (HPI);

- Review of systems (ROS); and

- Past, family and/or social history (PFSH).

The extent of history of present illness, review of systems, and past, family and/or social history that is obtained and documented is dependent upon clinical judgment and the nature of the presenting problem(s).

The chart below shows the progression of the elements required for each type of history. To qualify for a given type of history, **all three elements in the table must be met.** (A chief complaint is indicated at all levels.)

History of Present Illness (HPI)	Review of Systems (ROS)	Past, Family, and/or Social History (PFSH)	Type of History
Brief	N/A	N/A	Problem focused
Brief	Problem pertinent	N/A	Expanded problem focused
Extended	Extended	Pertinent	Detailed
Extended	Complete	Complete	Comprehensive

DG: The CC, ROS and PFSH may be listed as separate elements of history, or they may be included in the description of the history of the present illness.

DG: A ROS and/or a PFSH obtained during an earlier encounter does not need to be re-recorded if there is evidence that the physician reviewed and updated the previous information.

DG: This may occur when a physician updates his or her own record or in an institutional setting or group practice where many physicians use a common record. The review and update may be documented by:

- *describing any new ROS and/or PFSH information or noting there has been no change in the information; and*

- *noting the date and location of the earlier ROS and/or PFSH.*

DG: The ROS and/or PFSH may be recorded by ancillary staff or on a form completed by the patient. To document that the physician reviewed the information, there must be a notation supplementing or confirming the information recorded by others.

DG: If the physician is unable to obtain a history from the patient or other source, the record should describe the patient's condition or other circumstance which precludes obtaining a history.

Definitions and specific documentation guidelines for each of the elements of history are listed below.

Chief Complaint (CC)

The CC is a concise statement describing the symptom, problem, condition, diagnosis, physician recommended return, or other factor that is the reason for the encounter.

DG: The medical record should clearly reflect the chief complaint.

History of Present Illness (HPI)

The HPI is a chronological description of the development of the patient's present illness from the first sign and/or symptom or from the previous encounter to the present. It includes the following elements:

- location,
- quality,
- severity,
- duration,
- timing,
- context,
- modifying factors, and
- associated signs and symptoms.

Brief and *extended* HPIs are distinguished by the amount of detail needed to accurately characterize the clinical problem(s).

A *brief* HPI consists of one to three elements of the HPI.

DG: The medical record should describe one to three elements of the present illness (HPI).

An *extended* HPI consists of four or more elements of the HPI.

DG: The medical record should describe four or more elements of the present illness (HPI) or associated comorbidities.

Review of Systems (ROS)

A ROS is an inventory of body systems obtained through a series of questions seeking to identify signs and/or symptoms which the patient may be experiencing or has experienced.

For purposes of ROS, the following systems are recognized:

- Constitutional symptoms (e.g., fever, weight loss)
- Eyes
- Ears, Nose, Mouth, Throat
- Cardiovascular
- Respiratory
- Gastrointestinal
- Genitourinary
- Musculoskeletal
- Integumentary (skin and/or breast)
- Neurological
- Psychiatric
- Endocrine
- Hematologic/Lymphatic
- Allergic/Immunologic

A *problem pertinent* ROS inquires about the system directly related to the problem(s) identified in the HPI.

DG: The patient's positive responses and pertinent negatives for the system related to the problem should be documented.

An *extended* ROS inquires about the system directly related to the problem(s) identified in the HPI and a limited number of additional systems.

DG: The patient's positive responses and pertinent negatives for two to nine systems should be documented.

A *complete* ROS inquires about the system(s) directly related to the problem(s) identified in the HPI *plus* all additional body systems.

DG: At least ten organ systems must be reviewed. Those systems with positive or pertinent negative responses must be individually documented. For the remaining systems, a notation indicating all other systems are negative is permissible. In the absence of such a notation, at least ten systems must be individually documented.

Past, Family and/or Social History (PFSH)

The PFSH consists of a review of three areas:

- past history (the patient's past experiences with illnesses, operations, injuries and treatments);
- family history (a review of medical events in the patient's family, including diseases which may be hereditary or place the patient at risk); and
- social history (an age appropriate review of past and current activities).

For the categories of subsequent hospital care, follow-up inpatient consultations and subsequent nursing facility care, CPT requires only an "interval" history. It is not necessary to record information about the PFSH.

A *pertinent* PFSH is a review of the history area(s) directly related to the problem(s) identified in the HPI.

*DG: At least one specific item from **any** of the three history areas must be documented for a pertinent PFSH .*

A *complete* PFSH is of a review of two or all three of the PFSH history areas, depending on the category of the E/M service. A review of all three history areas is required for services that by their nature include a comprehensive assessment or reassessment of the patient. A review of two of the three history areas is sufficient for other services.

*DG: At least one specific item from **two** of the three history areas must be documented for a complete PFSH for the following categories of E/M services: office or other outpatient services, established patient; emergency department; subsequent nursing facility care; domiciliary care, established patient; and home care, established patient.*

*DG: At least one specific item from **each** of the three history areas must be documented for a complete PFSH for the following categories of E/M services: office or other outpatient services, new patient; hospital observation services; hospital inpatient services, initial care; consultations; comprehensive nursing facility assessments; domiciliary care, new patient; and homecare, new patient.*

B. Documentation of Examination

The levels of E/M services are based on four types of examination that are defined as follows:

- *Problem Focused*—a limited examination of the affected body area or organ system.
- *Expanded Problem Focused*—a limited examination of the affected body area or organ system and other symptomatic or related organ system(s).
- *Detailed*—an extended examination of the affected body area(s) and other symptomatic or related organ system(s).
- *Comprehensive*—a general multi-system examination or complete examination of a single organ system.

For purposes of examination, the following *body areas* are recognized:

- Head, including the face
- Neck
- Chest, including breasts and axillae
- Abdomen
- Genitalia, groin, buttocks
- Back, including spine
- Each extremity

For purposes of examination, the following *organ systems* are recognized:

- Constitutional (e.g., vital signs, general appearance)
- Eyes
- Ears, nose, mouth, and throat
- Cardiovascular
- Respiratory

- Gastrointestinal
- Genitourinary
- Musculoskeletal
- Skin
- Neurologic
- Psychiatric
- Hematologic/lymphatic/immunologic

The extent of examinations performed and documented is dependent upon clinical judgment and the nature of the presenting problem(s). They range from limited examinations of single body areas to general multi-system or complete single organ system examinations.

DG: Specific abnormal and relevant negative findings of the examination of the affected or symptomatic body area(s) or organ system(s) should be documented. A notation of "abnormal" without elaboration is insufficient.

DG: Abnormal or unexpected findings of the examination of the unaffected or asymptomatic body area(s) or organ system(s) should be described.

DG: A brief statement or notation indicating "negative" or "normal" is sufficient to document normal findings related to unaffected area(s) or asymptomatic organ system(s).

DG: The medical record for a general multi-system examination should include findings about 8 or more of the 12 organ systems.

C. Documentation of the Complexity of Medical Decision Making

The levels of E/M services recognize four types of medical decision making (straight-forward, low complexity, moderate complexity, and high complexity). Medical decision making refers to the complexity of establishing a diagnosis and/or selecting a management option as measured by:

- the number of possible diagnoses and/or the number of management options that must be considered;
- the amount and/or complexity of medical records, diagnostic tests, and/or other information that must be obtained, reviewed and analyzed; and
- the risk of significant complications, morbidity, and/or mortality, as well as comorbidities, associated with the patient's presenting problem(s), the diagnostic procedure(s) and/or the possible management options.

The chart below shows the progression of the elements required for each level of medical decision making. To qualify for a given type of decision making, **two of the three elements in the table must be either met or exceeded.**

Number of diagnoses or management options	Amount and/or complexity of data to be reviewed	Risk of complications and/or morbidity or mortality	Type of decision making
Minimal	Minimal or none	Minimal	Straightforward
Limited	Limited	Low	Low complexity
Multiple	Moderate	Moderate	Moderate complexity
Extensive	Extensive	High	High complexity

Each of the elements of medical decision making is described below.

Number of Diagnoses or Management Options

The number of possible diagnoses and/or the number of management options that must be considered is based on the number and types of problems addressed during the encounter, the complexity of establishing a diagnosis and the management decisions that are made by the physician.

Generally, decision making with respect to a diagnosed problem is easier than that for an identified but undiagnosed problem. The number and type of diagnostic tests employed may be an indicator of the number of possible diagnoses. Problems which are improving or resolving are less complex than those which are worsening or failing to change as expected. The need to seek advice from others is another indicator of complexity of diagnostic or management problems.

DG: For each encounter, an assessment, clinical impression, or diagnosis should be documented. It may be explicitly stated or implied in documented decisions regarding management plans and/or further evaluation.

- *For a presenting problem with an established diagnosis the record should reflect whether the problem is: a) improved, well controlled, resolving or resolved; or, b) inadequately controlled, worsening, or failing to change as expected.*

- *For a presenting problem without an established diagnosis, the assessment or clinical impression may be stated in the form of a differential diagnoses or as "possible," "probable," or "rule out" (R/O) diagnoses.*

DG: The initiation of, or changes in, treatment should be documented. Treatment includes a wide range of management options including patient instructions, nursing instructions, therapies, and medications.

DG: If referrals are made, consultations requested or advice sought, the record should indicate to whom or where the referral or consultation is made or from whom the advice is requested.

Amount and/or Complexity of Data to Be Reviewed

The amount and complexity of data to be reviewed is based on the types of diagnostic testing ordered or reviewed. A decision to obtain and review old medical records and/or obtain history from sources other than the patient increases the amount and complexity of data to be reviewed.

Discussion of contradictory or unexpected test results with the physician who performed or interpreted the test is an indication of the complexity of data being reviewed. On occasion the physician who ordered a test may personally review the image, tracing or specimen to supplement information from the physician who prepared the test report or interpretation; this is another indication of the complexity of data being reviewed.

DG: If a diagnostic service (test or procedure) is ordered, planned, scheduled, or performed at the time of the E/M encounter, the type of service, e.g., lab or x-ray, should be documented.

DG: The review of lab, radiology and/or other diagnostic tests should be documented. An entry in a progress note such as "WBC elevated" or "chest x-ray unremarkable" is acceptable. Alternatively, the review may be documented by initialing and dating the report containing the test results.

DG: A decision to obtain old records or decision to obtain additional history from the family, caretaker or other source to supplement that obtained from the patient should be documented.

DG: Relevant finding from the review of old records, and/or the receipt of additional history from the family, caretaker or other source should be documented. If there is no relevant information beyond that already obtained, that fact should be documented. A notation of "Old records reviewed" or "additional history obtained from family" without elaboration is insufficient.

DG: The results of discussion of laboratory, radiology or other diagnostic tests with the physician who performed or interpreted the study should be documented.

DG: The direct visualization and independent interpretation of an image, tracing, or specimen previously or subsequently interpreted by another physician should be documented.

Risk of Significant Complications, Morbidity, and/or Mortality

The risk of significant complications, morbidity, and/or mortality is based on the risks associated with the presenting problem(s), the diagnostic procedure(s), and the possible management options.

DG: Comorbidities/underlying diseases or other factors that increase the complexity of medical decision making by increasing the risk of complications, morbidity, and/or mortality should be documented.

DG: If a surgical or invasive diagnostic procedure is ordered, planned, or scheduled at the time of the E/M encounter, the type of procedure, e.g., laparoscopy, should be documented.

DG: If a surgical or invasive diagnostic procedure is performed at the time of the E/M encounter, the specific procedure should be documented.

DG: The referral for or decision to perform a surgical or invasive diagnostic procedure on an urgent basis should be documented or implied.

The following table may be used to help determine whether the risk of significant complications, morbidity, and/or mortality is *minimal*, *low*, *moderate*, or **high**. Because the determination of risk is complex and not readily quantifiable, the table includes common clinical examples rather than absolute measures of risk. The assessment of risk of the presenting problem(s) is based on the risk related to the disease process anticipated between the present encounter and the next one.

The assessment of risk of selecting diagnostic procedures and management options is based on the risk during and immediately following any procedures or treatment. The highest level of risk in any one category (presenting problem(s), diagnostic procedure(s), or management options) determines the overall risk.

Table of Risk

Level of risk	Presenting problem(s)	Diagnostic procedure(s) ordered	Management options selected
Minimal	One self-limiting or minor problem, e.g. cold, insect bite, tinea corporis	Laboratory tests requiring venipuncture Chest x-rays EKG/EEG Urinalysis Ultrasound, e.g., echocardiography KOH prep	Rest Gargles Elastic bandages Superficial dressings
Low	Two or more self-limiting or minor problems One stable chronic illness, e.g.,well controlled hypertension, non-insulin dependent diabetes, cataract, BPH Acute uncomplicated illness or injury, e.g., cystitis, allergic rhinitis, simple sprain	Physiologic tests not under stress, e.g., pulmonary function tests Non-cardiovascular imaging studies with contrast, e.g., barium enema Superficial needle biopsies Clinical laboratory tests requiring arterial puncture Skin biopsies	Over-the-counter drugs Minor surgery with no identified risk factors Physical therapy Occupational therapy IV fluids without additivies
Moderate	One or more chronic illnesses with mild exacerbation, progression, or side effects of treatment Two or more stable chronic illnesses Undiagnosed new problem with uncertain prognosis, e.g., lump in breast Acute illness with systemic symptoms, e.g., pyelonephritis, pneumonitis, colitis Acute complicated injury, e.g., head injury with brief loss of consciousness	Physiologic tests under stress, e.g., cardiac stress test, fetal contraction stress test Diagnostic endoscopies with no identified risk factors Deep needle or incisional biopsy Cardiovascular imaging studies with contrast and no identified risk factors, e.g., arteriogram, cardiac catheterization Obtain fluid from body cavity, e.g., lumbar puncture, thoracentesis, culdocentesis	Minor surgery with identified risk factors Elective major surgery (open, percutaneous, or endoscopic) with no identified risk factors Prescription drug management Therapeutic nuclear medicine IV fluids with additives Closed treatment of fracture or dislocation without manipulation
High	One or more chronic illnesses with severe exacerbation, progression, or side effects of treatment Acute or chronic illnesses or injuries that pose a threat to life or bodily function, e.g., multiple trauma, acute MI, pulmonary embolus, severe respiratory distress, progressive severe rheumatoid arthritis, psychiatric illness with potential threat to self or others, peritonitis, acute renal failure An abrupt change in neurologic status, e.g., seizure, TIA, weakness, or sensory loss	Cardiovascular imaging studies with contrast with identified risk factors Cardiac electrophysiological tests Diagnostic endoscopies with identified risk factors Discography	Elective major surgery (open, percutaneous, or endoscopic) with identified risk factors Emergency major surgery (open, percutaneous, or endoscopic) Parenteral controlled substances Drug therapy requiring intensive monitoring for toxicity Decision not to resuscitate or to de-escalate care because of poor prognosis

D. Documentation of an Encounter Dominated by Counseling or Coordination of Care

In the case where counseling and/or coordination of care dominates (more than 50%) of the physician/patient and/or family encounter (face-to-face time in the office or other outpatient setting or floor/unit time in the hospital or nursing facility), time is considered the key or controlling factor to qualify for a particular level of E/M services.

DG: If the physician elects to report the level of service based on counseling and/or coordination of care, the total length of time of the encounter (face-to-face or floor time, as appropriate) should be documented and the record should describe the counseling and/or activities to coordinate care.

B

1997 Documentation Guidelines for Evaluation and Management Services*

■ I. WHAT IS DOCUMENTATION AND WHY IS IT IMPORTANT?

Medical record documentation is required to record pertinent facts, findings, and observations about an individual's health history, including past and present illnesses, examinations, tests, treatments, and outcomes. The medical record chronologically documents the care of the patient and is an important element contributing to high-quality care. The medical record facilitates:

■ the ability of the physician and other health care professionals to evaluate and plan the patient's immediate treatment, and to monitor his/her health care over time;

■ communication and continuity of care among physicians and other health care professionals involved in the patient's care;

■ accurate and timely claims review and payment;

■ appropriate utilization review and quality of care evaluations; and

■ collection of data that may be useful for research and education.

An appropriately documented medical record can reduce many of the hassles associated with claims processing and may serve as a legal document to verify the care provided, if necessary.

■ WHAT DO PAYERS WANT AND WHY?

Because payers have a contractual obligation to enrollees, they may require reasonable documentation that services are consistent with the insurance coverage provided. They may request information to validate:

■ the site of service;

■ the medical necessity and appropriateness of the diagnostic and/or therapeutic services provided; and/or

■ that services provided have been accurately reported.

---

*Adapted from 1997 Documentation Guidelines For Evaluation and Management Services, Centers for Medicare & Medicaid Services, www.cms.gov/ (search "1997 documentation guidelines")

■ II. GENERAL PRINCIPLES OF MEDICAL RECORD DOCUMENTATION

The principles of documentation listed below are applicable to all types of medical and surgical services in all settings. For Evaluation and Management (E/M) services, the nature and amount of physician work and documentation varies by type of service, place of service, and the patient's status. The general principles listed below may be modified to account for these variable circumstances in providing E/M services.

1. The medical record should be complete and legible.

2. The documentation of each patient encounter should include:

   ■ reason for the encounter and relevant history, physical examination findings, and prior diagnostic test results;

   ■ assessment, clinical impression, or diagnosis;

   ■ plan for care; and

   ■ date and legible identity of the observer.

3. If not documented, the rationale for ordering diagnostic and other ancillary services should be easily inferred.

4. Past and present diagnoses should be accessible to the treating and/or consulting physician.

5. Appropriate health risk factors should be identified.

6. The patient's progress, response to and changes in treatment, and revision of diagnosis should be documented.

7. The CPT and ICD-9-CM codes reported on the health insurance claim form or billing statement should be supported by the documentation in the medical record.

■ III. DOCUMENTATION OF E/M SERVICES

This publication provides definitions and documentation guidelines for the three key components of E/M services and for visits that consist predominately of counseling or coordination of care. The three *key* components—history, examination, and medical decision-making—appear in the descriptors for office and other outpatient services, hospital observation services, hospital inpatient services, consultations, emergency department services, nursing facility services, domiciliary care services, and home services. While some of the text of CPT has been repeated in this publication, the reader should refer to CPT for the complete descriptors for E/M services and instructions for selecting a level of service. **Documentation guidelines are identified by the symbol *DG*.**

The descriptors for the levels of E/M services recognize seven components which are used in defining the levels of E/M services. These components are:

■ history;

■ examination;

■ medical decision making;

■ counseling;

■ coordination of care;

■ nature of presenting problem; and

■ time.

The first three of these components (i.e., history, examination, and medical decision making) are the key components in selecting the level of E/M services. In the case of visits that consist *predominantly* of counseling or coordination of care, time is the key or controlling factor to qualify for a particular level of E/M service.

Because the level of E/M service is dependent on two or three key components, performance and documentation of one component (e.g., examination) at the highest level does not necessarily mean that the encounter in its entirety qualifies for the highest level of E/M service.

These Documentation Guidelines for E/M services reflect the needs of the typical adult population. For certain groups of patients, the recorded information may vary slightly from that described here. Specifically, the medical records of infants, children, adolescents, and pregnant women may have additional or modified information recorded in each history and examination area.

As an example, newborn records may include under history of the present illness (HPI) the details of mother's pregnancy and the infant's status at birth; social history will focus on family structure; family history will focus on congenital anomalies and hereditary disorders in the family. In addition, the content of a pediatric examination will vary with the age and development of the child. Although not specifically defined in these documentation guidelines, these patient group variations on history and examination are appropriate.

A. Documentation of History

The levels of E/M services are based on four types of history (*problem focused, expanded problem focused, detailed,* and *comprehensive*). Each type of history includes some or all of the following elements:

- Chief complaint (CC)
- History of present illness (HPI)
- Review of systems (ROS)
- Past, family, and/or social history (PFSH)

The extent of history of present illness, review of systems, and past, family, and/or social history that is obtained and documented is dependent upon clinical judgment and the nature of the presenting problem(s).

The chart below shows the progression of the elements required for each type of history. To qualify for a given type of history, all three elements in the table must be met. (A chief complaint is indicated at all levels.)

History of Present Illness (HPI)	Review of Systems (ROS)	Past, Family, and/or Social History (PFSH)	Type of History
Brief	N/A	N/A	Problem focused
Brief	Problem pertinent	N/A	Expanded problem focused
Extended	Extended	Pertinent	Detailed
Extended	Complete	Complete	Comprehensive

DG: The CC, ROS, and PFSH may be listed as separate elements of history, or they may be included in the description of the history of the present illness.

DG: An ROS and/or a PFSH obtained during an earlier encounter does not need to be re-recorded if there is evidence that the physician reviewed and updated the previous information. This may occur when a physician updates his or her own record or in an institutional setting or group practice where many physicians use a common record. The review and update may be documented by:

- *describing any new ROS and/or PFSH information or noting there has been no change in the information; and*
- *noting the date and location of the earlier ROS and/or PFSH.*

DG: The ROS and/or PFSH may be recorded by ancillary staff or on a form completed by the patient. To document that the physician reviewed the information, there must be a notation supplementing or confirming the information recorded by others.

DG: If the physician is unable to obtain a history from the patient or other source, the record should describe the patient's condition or other circumstance that precludes obtaining a history.

Definitions and specific documentation guidelines for each of the elements of history are listed below.

Chief Complaint (CC)

The CC is a concise statement describing the symptom, problem, condition, diagnosis, physician recommended return, or other factor that is the reason for the encounter, usually stated in the patient's words. *DG: The medical record should clearly reflect the chief complaint.*

History of Present Illness (HPI)

The HPI is a chronological description of the development of the patient's present illness from the first sign and/or symptom or from the previous encounter to the present. It includes the following elements:

- location,
- quality,
- severity,
- duration,
- timing,
- context,
- modifying factors, and
- associated signs and symptoms.

Brief and *extended* HPIs are distinguished by the amount of detail needed to accurately characterize the clinical problem(s).

A *brief* HPI consists of one to three elements of the HPI.
DG: The medical record should describe one to three elements of the present illness (HPI).

An *extended* HPI consists of at least four elements of the HPI or the status of at least three chronic or inactive conditions.
DG: The medical record should describe at least four elements of the present illness (HPI), or the status of at least three chronic or inactive conditions.

Review of Systems (ROS)

An ROS is an inventory of body systems obtained through a series of questions seeking to identify signs and/or symptoms that the patient may be experiencing or has experienced. For purposes of ROS, the following systems are recognized:

- Constitutional symptoms (e.g., fever, weight loss)
- Eyes
- Ears, nose, mouth, throat
- Cardiovascular
- Respiratory
- Gastrointestinal
- Genitourinary
- Musculoskeletal
- Integumentary (skin and/or breast)
- Neurological
- Psychiatric
- Endocrine
- Hematologic/lymphatic
- Allergic/immunologic

A *problem-pertinent* ROS inquires about the system directly related to the problem(s) identified in the HPI.
DG: The patient's positive responses and pertinent negatives for the system related to the problem should be documented.

An *extended* ROS inquires about the system directly related to the problem(s) identified in the HPI and a limited number of additional systems.

DG: *The patient's positive responses and pertinent negatives for two to nine systems should be documented.*

A *complete* ROS inquires about the system(s) directly related to the problem(s) identified in the HPI *plus* all additional body systems.

DG: *At least ten organ systems must be reviewed. Those systems with positive or pertinent negative responses must be individually documented. For the remaining systems, a notation indicating all other systems are negative is permissible. In the absence of such a notation, at least ten systems must be individually documented.*

Past, Family, and/or Social History (PFSH)

The PFSH consists of a review of three areas:

■ Past history (the patient's past experiences with illnesses, operations, injuries, and treatments)

■ Family history (a review of medical events in the patient's family, including diseases that may be hereditary or place the patient at risk)

■ Social history (an age-appropriate review of past and current activities)

For certain categories of E/M services that include only an interval history, it is not necessary to record information about the PFSH. Those categories are subsequent hospital care, follow-up inpatient consultations, and subsequent nursing facility care.

A *pertinent* PFSH is a review of the history area(s) directly related to the problem(s) identified in the HPI.

DG: *At least one specific item from **any** of the three history areas must be documented for a pertinent PFSH.*

A *complete* PFSH is of a review of two or all three of the PFSH history areas, depending on the category of the E/M service. A review of all three history areas is required for services that by their nature include a comprehensive assessment or reassessment of the patient. A review of two of the three history areas is sufficient for other services.

DG: *At least one specific item from **two** of the three history areas must be documented for a complete PFSH for the following categories of E/M services: office or other outpatient services, established patient; emergency department; domiciliary care, established patient; and home care, established patient.*

DG: *At least one specific item from **each** of the three history areas must be documented for a complete PFSH for the following categories of E/M services: office or other outpatient services, new patient; hospital observation services; hospital inpatient services, initial care; consultations; comprehensive nursing facility assessments; domiciliary care, new patient; home care, new patient.*

B. Documentation of Examination

The levels of E/M services are based on four types of examination:

■ *Problem focused*—a limited examination of the affected body area or organ system.

■ *Expanded problem focused*—a limited examination of the affected body area or organ system and any other symptomatic or related body area(s) or organ system(s).

■ *Detailed*—an extended examination of the affected body area(s) or organ system(s) and any other symptomatic or related body area(s) or organ system(s).

■ *Comprehensive*—a general multisystem examination, or complete examination of a single organ system and other symptomatic or related body area(s) or organ system(s).

These types of examinations have been defined for general multisystem and the following single organ systems:

■ Cardiovascular

■ Ears, nose, mouth, and throat

■ Eyes

■ Genitourinary (female)

■ Genitourinary (male)

■ Hematologic/lymphatic/immunologic

- Musculoskeletal
- Neurological
- Psychiatric
- Respiratory
- Skin

A general multisystem examination or a single organ system examination may be performed by any physician regardless of specialty. The type (general multisystem or single organ system) and content of examination are selected by the examining physician and are based upon clinical judgment, the patient's history, and the nature of the presenting problem(s).

The content and documentation requirements for each type and level of examination are summarized below and described in detail in tables beginning on the next page. In the tables, organ systems and body areas recognized by CPT for purposes of describing examinations are shown in the left column. The content, or individual elements, of the examination pertaining to that body area or organ system are identified by bullets (•) in the right column.

Parenthetical examples—(e.g.,...)—have been used for clarification and to provide guidance regarding documentation. Documentation for each element must satisfy any numeric requirements (such as "Measurement of *any three of the following seven...*") included in the description of the element. Elements with multiple components but with no specific numeric requirement (such as "Examination of *liver* and *spleen*") require documentation of at least one component. It is possible for a given examination to be expanded beyond what is defined here. When that occurs, findings related to the additional systems and/or areas should be documented.

DG: Specific abnormal and relevant negative findings of the examination of the affected or symptomatic body area(s) or organ system(s) should be documented. A notation of "abnormal" without elaboration is insufficient.

DG: Abnormal or unexpected findings of the examination of any asymptomatic body area(s) or organ system(s) should be described.

DG: A brief statement or notation indicating "negative" or "normal" is sufficient to document normal findings related to unaffected area(s) or asymptomatic organ system(s).

GENERAL MULTISYSTEM EXAMINATIONS

General multisystem examinations are described in detail beginning on page 255. To qualify for a given level of multisystem examination, the following content and documentation requirements should be met:

- *Problem focused examination*—should include performance and documentation of one to five elements identified by a bullet (•) in one or more organ system(s) or body area(s).

- *Expanded problem focused examination*—should include performance and documentation of at least six elements identified by a bullet (•) in one or more organ system(s) or body area(s).

- *Detailed examination*—should include at least six organ systems or body areas. For each system/area selected, performance and documentation of at least two elements identified by a bullet (•) is expected. Alternatively, a detailed examination may include performance and documentation of at least twelve elements identified by a bullet (•) in two or more organ systems or body areas.

- *Comprehensive examination*—should include at least nine organ systems or body areas. For each system/area selected, all elements of the examination identified by a bullet (•) should be performed, unless specific directions limit the content of the examination. For each area/system, documentation of at least two elements identified by a bullet is expected.

SINGLE ORGAN SYSTEM EXAMINATIONS

The single organ system examinations recognized by CPT are described in detail beginning on page 255. Variations among these examinations in the organ systems and body areas identified in the left columns and in the elements of the examinations described in the right columns reflect differing emphases among specialties. To qualify for a given level of single organ system examination, the following content and documentation requirements should be met:

■ *Problem focused examination*—should include performance and documentation of one to five elements identified by a bullet (•), highlighted in bold or not.

■ *Expanded problem focused examination*—should include performance and documentation of at least six elements identified by a bullet (•), highlighted in bold or not.

■ *Detailed examination*—examinations other than the eye and psychiatric examinations should include performance and documentation of at least twelve elements identified by a bullet (•), highlighted in bold or not.

Eye and psychiatric examinations should include the performance and documentation of at least nine elements identified by a bullet (•), highlighted in bold or not.

■ *Comprehensive examination*—should include performance of all elements identified by a bullet (•), highlighted in bold or not. **Documentation of every element listed for each system/body area in *italics* and at least one element listed for other system/body areas is expected.**

Content and Documentation Requirements

General Multisystem Examination

System/Body Area	Elements of Examination
Constitutional	• Measurement of **any three of the following seven** vital signs: (1) sitting or standing blood pressure, (2) supine blood pressure, (3) pulse rate and regularity, (4) respiration, (5) temperature, (6) height, (7) weight (may be measured and recorded by ancillary staff) • General appearance of patient (e.g., development, nutrition, body habitus, deformities, attention to grooming)
Eyes	• Inspection of conjunctivae and lids • Examination of pupils and irises (e.g., reaction to light and accommodation, size and symmetry) • Ophthalmoscopic examination of optic discs (e.g., size, C/D ratio, appearance) and posterior segments (e.g., vessel changes, exudates, hemorrhages)
Ears, Nose, Mouth, and Throat	• External inspection of ears and nose (e.g., overall appearance, scars, lesions, masses) • Otoscopic examination of external auditory canals and tympanic membranes • Assessment of hearing (e.g., whispered voice, finger rub, tuning fork) • Inspection of nasal mucosa, septum, and turbinates • Inspection of lips, teeth, and gums • Examination of oropharynx: oral mucosa, salivary glands, hard and soft palates, tongue, tonsils, and posterior pharynx
Neck	• Examination of neck (e.g., masses, overall appearance, symmetry, tracheal position, crepitus) • Examination of thyroid (e.g., enlargement, tenderness, mass)
Respiratory	• Assessment of respiratory effort (e.g., intercostal retractions, use of accessory muscles, diaphragmatic movement) • Percussion of chest (e.g., dullness, flatness, hyperresonance) • Palpation of chest (e.g., tactile fremitus) • Auscultation of lungs (e.g., breath sounds, adventitious sounds, rubs)
Cardiovascular	• Palpation of heart (e.g., location, size, thrills) • Auscultation of heart with notation of abnormal sounds and murmurs Examination of: • Carotid arteries (e.g., pulse amplitude, bruits) • Abdominal aorta (e.g., size, bruits) • Femoral arteries (e.g., pulse amplitude, bruits) • Pedal pulses (e.g., pulse amplitude) • Extremities for edema and/or varicosities
Chest (Breasts)	• Inspection of breasts (e.g., symmetry, nipple discharge) • Palpation of breasts and axillae (e.g., masses or lumps, tenderness)

Continued

Content and Documentation Requirements—cont'd

General Multisystem Examination

System/Body Area	Elements of Examination
Gastrointestinal (Abdomen)	• Examination of abdomen with notation of presence of masses or tenderness • Examination of liver and spleen • Examination for presence or absence of hernia • Examination (when indicated) of anus, perineum, and rectum, including sphincter tone, presence of hemorrhoids, rectal masses • Obtain stool sample for occult blood test when indicated
Genitourinary	**MALE** • Examination of the scrotal contents (e.g., hydrocele, spermatocele, tenderness of cord, testicular mass) • Examination of the penis • Digital rectal examination of prostate gland (e.g., size, symmetry, nodularity, tenderness) **FEMALE** Pelvic examination (with or without specimen collection for smears and cultures), including: • Examination of external genitalia (e.g., general appearance, hair distribution, lesions) and vagina (e.g., general appearance, estrogen effect, discharge, lesions, pelvic support, cystocele, rectocele) • Examination of urethra (e.g., masses, tenderness, scarring) • Examination of bladder (e.g., fullness, masses, tenderness) • Cervix (e.g., general appearance, lesions, discharge) • Uterus (e.g., size, contour, position, mobility, tenderness, consistency, descent, or support) • Adnexa/parametria (e.g., masses, tenderness, organomegaly, nodularity)
Lymphatic	Palpation of lymph nodes in **two or more** areas: • Neck • Axillae • Groin • Other
Musculoskeletal	• Examination of gait and station • Inspection and/or palpation of digits and nails (e.g., clubbing, cyanosis, inflammatory conditions, petechiae, ischemia, infections, nodes) Examination of joints, bones, and muscles of **one or more of the following six areas:** (1) head and neck; (2) spine, ribs, and pelvis; (3) right upper extremity; (4) left upper extremity; (5) right lower extremity; and (6) left lower extremity. The examination of a given area includes: • Inspection and/or palpation with notation of presence of any misalignment, asymmetry, crepitation, defects, tenderness, masses, effusions • Assessment of range of motion with notation of any pain, crepitation, or contracture • Assessment of stability with notation of any dislocation (luxation), subluxation, or laxity • Assessment of muscle strength and tone (e.g., flaccid, cog wheel, spastic) with notation of any atrophy or abnormal movements
Skin	• Inspection of skin and subcutaneous tissue (e.g., rashes, lesions, ulcers) • Palpation of skin and subcutaneous tissue (e.g., induration, subcutaneous nodules, tightening)
Neurological	• Test cranial nerves with notation of any defects • Examination of deep tendon reflexes with notation of pathological reflexes (e.g., Babinski) • Examination of sensation (e.g., by touch, pin, vibration, proprioception)
Psychiatric	• Description of patient's judgment and insight Brief assessment of mental status, including: • Orientation to time, place, and person • Recent and remote memory • Mood and affect (e.g., depression, anxiety, agitation)

General Multisystem Content and Documentation Requirements

Level of Exam	Perform and Document
Problem focused	**One to five** elements identified by a bullet
Expanded problem focused	**At least six** elements identified by a bullet
Detailed	**At least two** elements identified by a bullet **from each of six areas/systems** OR **at least twelve** elements identified by a bullet in **two or more areas/systems**
Comprehensive	Perform **all elements** identified by a bullet in **at least nine** organ systems or body areas and document **at least two** elements identified by a bullet **from each of nine areas/systems**

Cardiovascular Examination

System/Body Area	Elements of Examination
Constitutional	• Measurement of **any three of the following seven** vital signs: (1) sitting or standing blood pressure, (2) supine blood pressure, (3) pulse rate and regularity, (4) respiration, (5) temperature, (6) height, (7) weight (may be measured and recorded by ancillary staff) • General appearance of patient (e.g., development, nutrition, body habitus, deformities, attention to grooming)
Eyes	• Inspection of conjunctivae and lids (e.g., xanthelasma)
Ears, Nose, Mouth, and Throat	• Inspection of teeth, gums, and palate • Examination of oral mucosa with notation of presence of pallor or cyanosis
Neck	• Examination of jugular veins (e.g., distention; a, v, or cannon a waves) • Examination of thyroid (e.g., enlargement, tenderness, mass)
Respiratory	• Assessment of respiratory effort (e.g., intercostal retractions, use of accessory muscles, diaphragmatic movement) • Auscultation of lungs (e.g., breath sounds, adventitious sounds, rubs)
Cardiovascular	• Palpation of heart (e.g., location, size, and forcefulness of the point of maximal impact; thrills; lifts; palpable S3 or S4) • Auscultation of heart, including sounds, abnormal sounds, and murmurs • Measurement of blood pressure in two or more extremities when indicated (e.g., aortic dissection, coarctation) Examination of: • Carotid arteries (e.g., waveform, pulse amplitude, bruits, apical-carotid delay) • Abdominal aorta (e.g., size, bruits) • Femoral arteries (e.g., pulse amplitude, bruits) • Pedal pulses (e.g., pulse amplitude) • Extremities for peripheral edema and/or varicosities
Gastrointestinal (Abdomen)	• Examination of abdomen with notation of presence of masses or tenderness • Examination of liver and spleen • Obtain stool sample for occult blood test from patients who are being considered for thrombolytic or anticoagulant therapy
Musculoskeletal	• Examination of the back with notation of kyphosis or scoliosis • Examination of gait with notation of ability to undergo exercise testing and/or participation in exercise programs • Assessment of muscle strength and tone (e.g., flaccid, cog wheel, spastic) with notation of any atrophy and abnormal movements
Extremities	• Inspection and palpation of digits and nails (e.g., clubbing, cyanosis, inflammation, petechiae, ischemia, infections, Osler's nodes)
Skin	• Inspection and/or palpation of skin and subcutaneous tissue (e.g., stasis dermatitis, ulcers, scars, xanthomas)
Neurological/ Psychiatric	Brief assessment of mental status, including: • Orientation to time, place, and person • Mood and affect (e.g., depression, anxiety, agitation)

Cardiovascular Content and Documentation Requirements

Level of Exam	Perform and Document
Problem focused	**One to five** elements identified by a bullet
Expanded problem focused	**At least six** elements identified by a bullet
Detailed	**At least twelve** elements identified by a bullet
Comprehensive	Perform **all elements** identified by a bullet; document every element in *italics* and at least one non-italicized element in each section

Ear, Nose, and Throat Examination

System/Body Area	Elements of Examination
Constitutional	• Measurement of **any three of the following seven** vital signs: (1) sitting or standing blood pressure, (2) supine blood pressure, (3) pulse rate and regularity, (4) respiration, (5) temperature, (6) height, (7) weight (may be measured and recorded by ancillary staff) • General appearance of patient (e.g., development, nutrition, body habitus, deformities, attention to grooming) • Assessment of ability to communicate (e.g., use of sign language or other communication aids) and quality of voice
Head and Face	• Inspection of head and face (e.g., overall appearance, scars, lesions, and masses) • Palpation and/or percussion of face with notation of presence or absence of sinus tenderness • Examination of salivary glands • Assessment of facial strength
Eyes	• Test ocular motility, including primary gaze alignment
Ears, Nose, Mouth, and Throat	• Otoscopic examination of external auditory canals and tympanic membranes, including pneumo-otoscopy with notation of mobility of membranes • Assessment of hearing with tuning forks and clinical speech reception thresholds (e.g., whispered voice, finger rub) • External inspection of ears and nose (e.g., overall appearance, scars, lesions, and masses) • Inspection of nasal mucosa, septum, and turbinates • Inspection of lips, teeth, and gums • Examination of oropharynx: oral mucosa, salivary glands, hard and soft palates, tongue, tonsils, and posterior pharynx (e.g., asymmetry, lesions, hydration of mucosal surfaces) • Inspection of pharyngeal walls and pyriform sinuses (e.g., pooling of saliva, asymmetry, lesions) • Examination by mirror of larynx, including the condition of the epiglottis, false vocal cords, true vocal cords, and mobility of larynx (use of mirror not required in children) • Examination by mirror of nasopharynx, including appearance of mucosa, adenoids, posterior choanae, and eustachian tubes (use of mirror not required in children)
Neck	• Examination of neck (e.g., masses, overall appearance, symmetry, tracheal position, crepitus) • Examination of thyroid (e.g., enlargement, tenderness, mass)
Respiratory	• Inspection of chest, including symmetry, expansion, and/or assessment of respiratory effort (e.g., intercostal retractions, use of accessory muscles, diaphragmatic movement) • Auscultation of lungs (e.g., breath sounds, adventitious sounds, rubs)
Cardiovascular	• Auscultation of heart with notation of abnormal sounds and murmurs • Examination of peripheral vascular system by observation (e.g., swelling, varicosities) and palpation (e.g., pulse, temperature, edema, tenderness)
Lymphatic	Palpation of lymph nodes in neck, axillae, groin, or other region
Neurological/ Psychiatric	• Test cranial nerves with notation of any defects Brief assessment of mental status, including: • Orientation to time, place, and person • Mood and affect (e.g., depression, anxiety, agitation)

Ear, Nose, and Throat Content and Documentation Requirements

Level of Exam	Perform and Document
Problem focused	**One to five** elements identified by a bullet
Expanded problem focused	**At least six** elements identified by a bullet
Detailed	**At least two** elements identified by a bullet
Comprehensive	Perform **all elements** identified by a bullet; document every element in **bold** and at least one non-bold element in each section

Eye Examination

System/Body Area	Elements of Examination
Eyes	• Test visual acuity (Does not include determination of refractive error) • Gross visual field testing by confrontation • Test ocular motility, including primary gaze alignment • Examination of ocular adnexa, including lids (e.g., ptosis or lagophthalmos), lacrimal glands, lacrimal drainage, orbits, and preauricular lymph nodes • Examination of pupils and irises, including shape, direct and consensual reaction (afferent pupil), size (e.g., anisocoria), and morphology • Slit lamp examination of the corneas, including epithelium, stroma, endothelium, and tear film • Slit lamp examination of the anterior chambers, including depth, cells, and flare • Slit lamp examination of the lenses, including clarity, anterior and posterior capsule, cortex, and nucleus • Measurement of intraocular pressures (except in children and patients with trauma or infectious disease) Ophthalmoscopic examination through dilated pupils (unless contraindicated) of • Optic discs, including size, C/D ratio, appearance (e.g., atrophy, cupping, tumor elevation) and nerve fiber layer • Posterior segments, including retina and vessels (e.g., exudates and hemorrhages)
Neurological/ Psychiatric	Brief assessment of mental status, including: • Orientation to time, place, and person • Mood and affect (e.g., depression, anxiety, agitation)

Eye Content and Documentation Requirements

Level of Exam	Perform and Document
Problem focused	**One to five** elements identified by a bullet
Expanded problem focused	**At least six** elements identified by a bullet
Detailed	**At least nine** elements identified by a bullet
Comprehensive	Perform **all elements** identified by a bullet; document every element in *italics* and at least one non-italicized element in each section

Genitourinary Examination

System/Body Area	Elements of Examination
Constitutional	• Measurement of **any three of the following seven** vital signs: (1) sitting or standing blood pressure, (2) supine blood pressure, (3) pulse rate and regularity, (4) respiration, (5) temperature, (6) height, (7) weight (may be measured and recorded by ancillary staff) • General appearance of patient (e.g., development, nutrition, body habitus, deformities, attention to grooming)
Neck	• Examination of neck (e.g., masses, overall appearance, symmetry, tracheal position, crepitus) • Examination of thyroid (e.g., enlargement, tenderness, mass)
Respiratory	• Assessment of respiratory effort (e.g., intercostal retractions, use of accessory muscles, diaphragmatic movement) • Auscultation of lungs (e.g., breath sounds, adventitious sounds, rubs)
Cardiovascular	• Auscultation of heart with notation of abnormal sounds and murmurs • Examination of peripheral vascular system by observation (e.g., swelling, varicosities) and palpation (e.g., pulse, temperature, edema, tenderness)
Chest (Breasts)	(See genitourinary [female])
Gastrointestinal (Abdomen)	• Examination of abdomen with notation of presence of masses or tenderness • Examination for presence or absence of hernia • Examination of liver and spleen • Obtain stool sample for occult blood test when indicated
Genitourinary	**MALE** • Inspection of anus and perineum Examination (with or without specimen collection for smears and cultures) of genitalia, including: • Scrotum (e.g., lesions, cysts, rashes) • Epididymides (e.g., size, symmetry, masses) • Testes (e.g., size, symmetry, masses) • Urethral meatus (e.g., size, location, lesions, discharge) • Penis (e.g., lesions, presence or absence of foreskin, foreskin retractability, plaque, masses, scarring, deformities) Digital rectal examination, including: • Prostate gland (e.g., size, symmetry, nodularity, tenderness) • Seminal vesicles (e.g., symmetry, tenderness, masses, enlargement) • Sphincter tone, presence of hemorrhoids, rectal masses **FEMALE** Include **at least seven of the following eleven** elements identified by bullets: • Inspection and palpation of breasts (e.g., masses or lumps, tenderness, symmetry, nipple discharge) • Digital rectal examination, including sphincter tone, presence of hemorrhoids, rectal masses Pelvic examination (with or without specimen collection for smears and cultures), including: • External genitalia (e.g., general appearance, hair distribution, lesions) • Urethral meatus (e.g., size, location, lesions, prolapse) • Urethra (e.g., masses, tenderness, scarring) • Bladder (e.g., fullness, masses, tenderness) • Vagina (e.g., general appearance, estrogen effect, discharge, lesions, pelvic support, cystocele, rectocele) • Cervix (e.g., general appearance, lesions, discharge) • Uterus (e.g., size, contour, position, mobility, tenderness, consistency, descent or support) • Adnexa/parametria (e.g., masses, tenderness, organomegaly, nodularity) • Anus and perineum • Palpation of lymph nodes in neck, axillae, groin, or other region
Skin	• Inspection and/or palpation of skin and subcutaneous tissue (e.g., rashes, lesions, ulcers)
Neurological/ Psychiatric	Brief assessment of mental status, including: • Orientation (such as to time, place, and person) • Mood and affect (e.g., depression, anxiety, agitation)

Genitourinary Content and Documentation Requirements

Level of Exam	Perform and Document
Problem focused	**One to five** elements identified by a bullet
Expanded problem focused	**At least six** elements identified by a bullet
Detailed	**At least twelve** elements identified by a bullet
Comprehensive	Perform **all elements** identified by a bullet; document every element in **bold** and at least one non-bold element in each section

Hematologic/Lymphatic/Immunologic Examination

System/Body Area	Elements of Examination
Constitutional	• Measurement of **any three of the following seven** vital signs: (1) sitting or standing blood pressure, (2) supine blood pressure, (3) pulse rate and regularity, (4) respiration, (5) temperature, (6) height, (7) weight (may be measured and recorded by ancillary staff) • General appearance of patient (e.g., development, nutrition, body habitus, deformities, attention to grooming)
Head and Face	• Palpation and/or percussion of face with notation of presence or absence of sinus tenderness
Eyes	• Inspection of conjunctivae and lids
Ears, Nose, Mouth, and Throat	• Otoscopic examination of external auditory canals and tympanic membranes • Inspection of nasal mucosa, septum, and turbinates • Inspection of teeth and gums • Examination of oropharynx (e.g., oral mucosa, hard and soft palates, tongue, tonsils, and posterior pharynx)
Neck	• Examination of neck (e.g., masses, overall appearance, symmetry, tracheal position, crepitus) • Examination of thyroid (e.g., enlargement, tenderness, mass)
Respiratory	• Assessment of respiratory effort (e.g., intercostal retractions, use of accessory muscles, diaphragmatic movement) • Auscultation of lungs (e.g., breath sounds, adventitious sounds, rubs)
Cardiovascular	• Auscultation of heart with notation of abnormal sounds and murmurs • Examination of peripheral vascular system by observation (e.g., swelling, varicosities) and palpation (e.g., pulses, temperature, edema, tenderness)
Gastrointestinal (Abdomen)	• Examination of abdomen with notation of presence of masses or tenderness • Examination of liver and spleen
Lymphatic	• Palpation of lymph nodes in neck, axillae, groin, or other region
Extremities	• Inspection and palpation of digits and nails (e.g., clubbing, cyanosis, inflammation, petechiae, ischemia, infections, Osler's nodes)
Skin	• Inspection and/or palpation of skin and subcutaneous tissue (e.g., rashes, lesions, ulcers, ecchymoses, bruises)
Neurological/ Psychiatric	Brief assessment of mental status, including: • Orientation to time, place, and person • Mood and affect (e.g., depression, anxiety, agitation)

Hematologic/Lymphatic/Immunologic Content and Documentation Requirements

Level of Exam	Perform and Document
Problem focused	**One to five** elements identified by a bullet
Expanded problem focused	**At least six** elements identified by a bullet
Detailed	**At least twelve** elements identified by a bullet
Comprehensive	Perform **all elements** identified by a bullet; document every element in **bold** and at least one non-bold element in each section

Musculoskeletal Examination

System/Body Area	Elements of Examination
Constitutional	• Measurement of **any three of the following seven** vital signs: (1) sitting or standing blood pressure, (2) supine blood pressure, (3) pulse rate and regularity, (4) respiration, (5) temperature, (6) height, (7) weight (may be measured and recorded by ancillary staff) • General appearance of patient (e.g., development, nutrition, body habitus, deformities, attention to grooming)
Cardiovascular	• Examination peripheral vascular system by observation (e.g., swelling, varicosities) and palpation (e.g., pulses, temperature, edema, tenderness)
Lymphatic	• Palpation of lymph nodes in neck, axillae, groin, or other region
Musculoskeletal	• Examination of gait and station
	Examination of joints, bones, and muscles/tendons of **four of the following six** areas: (1) head and neck; (2) spine, ribs, and pelvis; (3) right upper extremity; (4) left upper extremity; (5) right lower extremity; and (6) left lower extremity. The examination of a given area includes:
	• Inspection, percussion, and/or palpation with notation of any misalignment, asymmetry, crepitation, defects, tenderness, masses, or effusions • Assessment of range of motion with notation of any pain (e.g., straight leg raising), crepitation, or contracture • Assessment of stability with notation of any dislocation (luxation), subluxation, or laxity • Assessment of muscle strength and tone (e.g., flaccid, cog wheel, spastic) with notation of any atrophy or abnormal movements
	NOTE: For the comprehensive level of examination, all four of the elements identified by a bullet must be performed and documented for each of four anatomic areas. For the three lower levels of examination, each element is counted separately for each body area. For example, assessing range of motion in two extremities constitutes two elements. (See musculoskeletal and skin)
Extremities	
Skin	• Inspection and/or palpation of skin and subcutaneous tissue (e.g., scars, rashes, lesions, café-au-lait spots, ulcers) in **four of the following six** areas: (1) head and neck, (2) trunk, (3) right upper extremity, (4) left upper extremity, (5) right lower extremity, and (6) left lower extremity.
	NOTE: For the comprehensive level, all four anatomic areas must be performed and documented. For the three lower levels of examination, each body area is counted separately. For example, inspection and/or palpation of skin and subcutaneous tissue in two extremities constitutes two elements.
Neurological/ Psychiatric	• Test coordination (e.g., finger/nose, heel/knee/shin, rapid alternating movements in the upper and lower extremities, evaluation of the fine motor coordination in young children) • Examination of deep tendon reflexes and/or nerve stretch test with notation of pathological reflexes (e.g., Babinski) • Examination of sensation (e.g., by touch, pin, vibration, proprioception)
	Brief assessment of mental status, including:
	• Orientation to time, place, and person • Mood and affect (e.g., depression, anxiety, agitation)

Musculoskeletal Content and Documentation Requirements

Level of Exam	Perform and Document
Problem focused	**One to five** elements identified by a bullet
Expanded problem focused	**At least six** elements identified by a bullet
Detailed	**At least twelve** elements identified by a bullet
Comprehensive	Perform **all elements** identified by a bullet; document every element in **bold** and at least one non-bold element in each section

Neurological Examination	
System/Body Area	**Elements of Examination**
Constitutional	• Measurement of **any three of the following seven** vital signs: (1) sitting or standing blood pressure, (2) supine blood pressure, (3) pulse rate and regularity, (4) respiration, (5) temperature, (6) height, (7) weight (may be measured and recorded by ancillary staff)
	• General appearance of patient (e.g., development, nutrition, body habitus, deformities, attention to grooming)
Eyes	• Ophthalmoscopic examination of optic discs (e.g., size, C/D ratio, appearance) and posterior segments (e.g., vessel changes, exudates, hemorrhages)
Cardiovascular	• Examination of carotid arteries (e.g., pulse amplitude, bruits)
	• Auscultation of heart with notation of abnormal sounds and murmurs
	• Examination of peripheral vascular system by observation (e.g., swelling, varicosities) and palpation (e.g., pulses, temperature, edema, tenderness)
Musculoskeletal	• Examination of gait and station
	Assessment of motor function, including:
	• Muscle strength in upper and lower extremities
	• Muscle tone in upper and lower extremities (e.g., flaccid, cog wheel, spastic) with notation of atrophy or abnormal movements (e.g., fasciculation, tardive dyskinesia)
Extremities	(See musculoskeletal)
Neurological	Evaluation of higher integrative functions, including:
	• Orientation to time, place, and person
	• Recent and remote memory
	• Attention span and concentration
	• Language (e.g., naming objects, repeating phrases, spontaneous speech)
	• Fund of knowledge (e.g., awareness of current events, past history, vocabulary)
	Test the following cranial nerves:
	• 2nd cranial nerve (e.g., visual acuity, visual fields, fundi)
	• 3rd, 4th, and 6th cranial nerves (e.g., pupils, eye movements)
	• 5th cranial nerve (e.g., facial sensation, corneal reflex)
	• 7th cranial nerve (e.g., facial symmetry, strength)
	• 8th cranial nerve (e.g., hearing with tuning fork, whispered voice, and/or finger rub)
	• 9th cranial nerve (e.g., spontaneous or reflex palate movement)
	• 11th cranial nerve (e.g., shoulder shrug strength)
	• 12th cranial nerve (e.g., tongue protrusion)
	• Examination of sensation (e.g., by touch, pin, vibration, proprioception)
	• Examination of deep tendon reflexes with notation of pathologic reflexes (e.g., Babinski)
	• Test coordination (e.g., finger/nose, heel/knee/shin, rapid alternating movements in the upper and lower extremities, evaluation of the fine motor coordination in young children)

Neurological Content and Documentation Requirements	
Level of Exam	**Perform and Document**
Problem focused	**One to five** elements identified by a bullet
Expanded problem focused	**At least six** elements identified by a bullet
Detailed	**At least twelve** elements identified by a bullet
Comprehensive	Perform **all** elements identified by a bullet; document every element in **bold** and at least one non-bold element in each section

Psychiatric Examination

System/Body Area	Elements of Examination
Constitutional	• Measurement of **any three of the following seven** vital signs: (1) sitting or standing blood pressure, (2) supine blood pressure, (3) pulse rate and regularity, (4) respiration, (5) temperature, (6) height, (7) weight (may be measured and recorded by ancillary staff) • General appearance of patient (e.g., development, nutrition, body habitus, deformities, attention to grooming)
Musculoskeletal	• Assessment of muscle strength and tone (e.g., flaccid, cog wheel, spastic) with notation of any atrophy or abnormal movements • Examination of gait and station
Psychiatric	• Description of speech, including rate, volume, articulation, coherence, and spontaneity with notation of abnormalities (e.g., perseveration, paucity of language) • Description of thought processes, including rate of thoughts, content of thoughts (e.g., logical vs. illogical, tangential), abstract reasoning, and computation • Description of associations (e.g., loose, tangential, circumstantial, intact) • Description of abnormal or psychotic thoughts, including hallucinations, delusions, preoccupation with violence, homicidal or suicidal ideation, and obsessions • Description of the patient's judgment (e.g., concerning everyday activities and social situations) and insight (e.g., concerning psychiatric condition) Complete mental status examination, including: • Orientation to time, place, and person • Recent and remote memory • Attention span and concentration • Language (e.g., naming objects, repeating phrases) • Fund of knowledge (e.g., awareness of current events, past history, vocabulary) • Mood and affect (e.g., depression, anxiety, agitation, hypomania, lability) Brief assessment of mental status, including: • Orientation to time, place, and person • Recent and remote memory • Mood and affect (e.g., depression, anxiety, agitation)

Psychiatric Content and Documentation Requirements

Level of Exam	Perform and Document
Problem focused	**One to five** elements identified by a bullet
Expanded problem focused	**At least six** elements identified by a bullet
Detailed	**At least nine** elements identified by a bullet
Comprehensive	Perform **all elements** identified by a bullet; document every element in **bold** and at least one non-bold element in each section

Respiratory Examination

System/Body Area	Elements of Examination
Constitutional	• Measurement of **any three of the following seven** vital signs: (1) sitting or standing blood pressure, (2) supine blood pressure, (3) pulse rate and regularity, (4) respiration, (5) temperature, (6) height, (7) weight (may be measured and recorded by ancillary staff) • General appearance of patient (e.g., development, nutrition, body habitus, deformities, attention to grooming)
Ears, Nose, Mouth, and Throat	• Inspection of nasal mucosa, septum, and turbinates • Inspection of teeth and gums • Examination of oropharynx (e.g., oral mucosa, hard and soft palates, tongue, tonsils, and posterior pharynx)
Neck	• Examination of neck (e.g., masses, overall appearance, symmetry, tracheal position, crepitus) • Examination of thyroid (e.g., enlargement, tenderness, mass) • Examination of jugular veins (e.g., distention, a, v, or cannon waves)
Respiratory	• Inspection of chest with notation of symmetry and expansion • Assessment of respiratory effort (e.g., intercostal retractions, use of accessory muscles, diaphragmatic movement) • Percussion of chest (e.g., dullness, flatness, hyperresonance) • Palpation of chest (e.g., tactile fremitus) • Auscultation of lungs (e.g., breath sounds, adventitious sounds, rubs)
Cardiovascular	• Auscultation of heart, with notation of abnormal sounds and murmurs • Examination of peripheral vascular system by observation (e.g., swelling, varicosities) and palpation (e.g., pulses, temperature, edema, tenderness)
Gastrointestinal (Abdomen)	• Examination of abdomen with notation of presence of masses or tenderness • Examination of liver and spleen
Lymphatic	• Palpation of lymph nodes in neck, axillae, groin, and/or other location
Musculoskeletal	• Assessment of muscle strength and tone (e.g., flaccid, cog wheel, spastic) with notation of any atrophy or abnormal movements • Examination of gait and station
Extremities	• Inspection and palpation of digits and nails (e.g., clubbing, cyanosis, inflammation, petechiae, ischemia, infections, nodes)
Skin	• Inspection and/or palpation of skin and subcutaneous tissue (e.g., rashes, lesions, ulcers)
Neurological/ Psychiatric	Brief assessment of mental status, including: • Orientation to time, place, and person • Mood and affect (e.g., depression, anxiety, agitation)

Respiratory Content and Documentation Requirements

Level of Exam	Perform and Document
Problem focused	**One to five** elements identified by a bullet
Expanded problem focused	**At least six** elements identified by a bullet
Detailed	**At least twelve** elements identified by a bullet
Comprehensive	Perform **all elements** identified by a bullet; document every element in **bold** and at least one non-bold element in each section

Skin Examination

System/Body Area	Elements of Examination
Constitutional	• Measurement of **any three of the following seven** vital signs: (1) sitting or standing blood pressure, (2) supine blood pressure, (3) pulse rate and regularity, (4) respiration, (5) temperature, (6) height, (7) weight (may be measured and recorded by ancillary staff) • General appearance of patient (e.g., development, nutrition, body habitus, deformities, attention to grooming)
Eyes	• Inspection of conjunctivae and lids
Ears, Nose, Mouth, and Throat	• Inspection of lips, teeth, and gums • Examination of oropharynx (e.g., oral mucosa, hard and soft palates, tongue, tonsils, posterior pharynx)
Neck	• Examination of thyroid (e.g., enlargement, tenderness, mass)
Cardiovascular	• Examination of peripheral vascular system by observation (e.g., swelling, varicosities) and palpation (e.g., pulses, temperature, edema, tenderness)
Chest (Breasts)	
Gastrointestinal (Abdomen)	• Examination of liver and spleen • Examination of anus for condyloma and other lesions
Lymphatic	• Palpation of lymph nodes in neck, axillae, groin, and/or other location
Extremities	• Inspection and palpation of digits and nails (e.g., clubbing, cyanosis, inflammation, petechiae, ischemia, infections, nodes)
Skin	• Palpation of scalp and inspection of hair of scalp, eyebrows, face, chest, pubic area (when indicated), and extremities • Inspection and/or palpation of skin and subcutaneous tissue (e.g., rashes, lesions, ulcers, susceptibility to and presence of photo damage) in **eight of the following ten** areas: • Head, including the face • Neck • Chest, including breasts and axillae • Abdomen • Genitalia, groin, buttocks • Back • Right upper extremity • Left upper extremity • Right lower extremity • Left lower extremity **NOTE:** For the comprehensive level, the examination of at least eight anatomic areas must be performed and documented. For the three lower levels of examination, each body area is counted separately. For example, inspection and/or palpation of the skin and subcutaneous tissue of the right upper extremity and the left upper extremity constitute two elements. • Inspection of eccrine and apocrine glands of the skin and subcutaneous tissue with identification of any hyperhidrosis, chromhidroses, or bromhidrosis
Neurological/ Psychiatric	Brief assessment of mental status, including: • Orientation to time, place, and person • Mood and affect (e.g., depression, anxiety, agitation)

Skin Content and Documentation Requirements

Level of Exam	Perform and Document
Problem focused	**One to five** elements identified by a bullet
Expanded problem focused	**At least six** elements identified by a bullet
Detailed	**At least twelve** elements identified by a bullet
Comprehensive	Perform **all elements** identified by a bullet; document every element in **bold** and at least one non-bold element in each section

C. Documentation of the Complexity of Medical Decision-Making

The levels of E/M services recognize four types of medical decision-making (straightforward, low complexity, moderate complexity, and high complexity). Medical decision-making refers to the complexity of establishing a diagnosis and/or selecting a management option as measured by:

■ the number of possible diagnoses and/or the number of management options that must be considered;

■ the amount and/or complexity of medical records, diagnostic tests, and/or other information that must be obtained, reviewed, and analyzed; and

■ the risk of significant complications, morbidity and/or mortality, as well as comorbidities, associated with the patient's presenting problem(s), the diagnostic procedure(s), and/or the possible management options.

   The chart below shows the progression of the elements required for each level of medical decision-making. To qualify for a given type of decision-making, **two of the three elements in the table must be either met or exceeded.**

Number of diagnoses or management options	Amount and/or complexity of data to be reviewed	Risk of complications and/or morbidity or mortality	Type of decision making
Minimal	Minimal or none	Minimal	Straightforward
Limited	Limited	Low	Low complexity
Multiple	Moderate	Moderate	Moderate complexity
Extensive	Extensive	High	High complexity

   Each of the elements of medical decision-making is described below.

■ NUMBER OF DIAGNOSES OR MANAGEMENT OPTIONS

The number of possible diagnoses and/or the number of management options that must be considered is based on the number and types of problems addressed during the encounter, the complexity of establishing a diagnosis, and the management decisions that are made by the physician.

   Generally, decision-making with respect to a diagnosed problem is easier than that for an identified but undiagnosed problem. The number and type of diagnostic tests employed may be an indicator of the number of possible diagnoses. Problems that are improving or resolving are less complex than those that are worsening or failing to change as expected. The need to seek advice from others is another indicator of complexity of diagnostic or management problems.

DG: For each encounter, an assessment, clinical impression, or diagnosis should be documented. It may be explicitly stated or implied in documented decisions regarding management plans and/or further evaluation.

■ *For a presenting problem with an established diagnosis, the record should reflect whether the problem is (a) improved, well controlled, resolving, or resolved or (b) inadequately controlled, worsening, or failing to change as expected.*

■ *For a presenting problem without an established diagnosis, the assessment or clinical impression may be stated in the form of differential diagnoses or as a "possible," "probable," or "rule out" (R/O) diagnosis.*

DG: The initiation of, or changes in, treatment should be documented. Treatment includes a wide range of management options, including patient instructions, nursing instructions, therapies, and medications.

DG: If referrals are made, consultations requested or advice sought, the record should indicate to whom or where the referral or consultation is made or from whom the advice is requested.

■ AMOUNT AND/OR COMPLEXITY OF DATA TO BE REVIEWED

The amount and complexity of data to be reviewed is based on the types of diagnostic testing ordered or reviewed. A decision to obtain and review old medical records and/or obtain history from sources other than the patient increases the amount and complexity of data to be reviewed.

Discussion of contradictory or unexpected test results with the physician who performed or interpreted the test is an indication of the complexity of data being reviewed. On occasion the physician who ordered a test may personally review the image, tracing, or specimen to supplement information from the physician who prepared the test report or interpretation; this is another indication of the complexity of data being reviewed.

DG: If a diagnostic service (test or procedure) is ordered, planned, scheduled, or performed at the time of the E/M encounter, the type of service (e.g., lab or x-ray) should be documented.

DG: The review of lab, radiology, and/or other diagnostic tests should be documented. A simple notation such as "WBC elevated" or "chest x-ray unremarkable" is acceptable. Alternatively, the review may be documented by initialing and dating the report containing the test results.

DG: A decision to obtain old records or a decision to obtain additional history from the family, caretaker, or other source to supplement that obtained from the patient should be documented.

DG: Relevant findings from the review of old records, and/or the receipt of additional history from the family, caretaker, or other source to supplement that obtained from the patient should be documented. If there is no relevant information beyond that already obtained, that fact should be documented. A notation of "Old records reviewed" or "Additional history obtained from family" without elaboration is insufficient.

DG: The results of discussion of laboratory, radiology, or other diagnostic tests with the physician who performed or interpreted the study should be documented.

DG: The direct visualization and independent interpretation of an image, tracing, or specimen previously or subsequently interpreted by another physician should be documented.

■ RISK OF SIGNIFICANT COMPLICATIONS, MORBIDITY, AND/OR MORTALITY

The risk of significant complications, morbidity, and/or mortality is based on the risks associated with the presenting problem(s), the diagnostic procedure(s), and the possible management options.

DG: Comorbidities/underlying diseases or other factors that increase the complexity of medical decision-making by increasing the risk of complications, morbidity, and/or mortality should be documented.

DG: If a surgical or invasive diagnostic procedure is ordered, planned, or scheduled at the time of the E/M encounter, the type of procedure (e.g., laparoscopy) should be documented.

DG: If a surgical or invasive diagnostic procedure is performed at the time of the E/M encounter, the specific procedure should be documented.

DG: The referral for or decision to perform a surgical or invasive diagnostic procedure on an urgent basis should be documented or implied.

The following table may be used to help determine whether the risk of significant complications, morbidity, and/or mortality is *minimal*, *low*, *moderate*, or *high*. Because the determination of risk is complex and not readily quantifiable, the table includes common clinical examples rather than absolute measures of risk. The assessment of risk of the presenting problem(s) is based on the risk related to the disease process anticipated between the present encounter and the next one. The assessment of risk of selecting diagnostic procedures and management options is based on the risk during and immediately following any procedure or treatment. **The highest level of risk in any one category (presenting problem[s], diagnostic procedure[s], or management options) determines the overall risk.**

Table of Risk

Level of risk	Presenting problem(s)	Diagnostic procedure(s) ordered	Management options selected
Minimal	One self-limiting or minor problem (e.g., cold, insect bite, tinea corporis)	Laboratory tests requiring venipuncture Chest x-rays EKG/EEG Urinalysis Ultrasound (e.g., echocardiography) KOH prep	Rest Gargles Elastic bandages Superficial dressings
Low	Two or more self-limiting or minor problems One stable chronic illness (e.g., well-controlled hypertension, non-insulin-dependent diabetes, cataract, BPH) Acute uncomplicated illness or injury (e.g., cystitis, allergic rhinitis, simple sprain)	Physiologic tests not under stress (e.g., pulmonary function tests) Non-cardiovascular imaging studies with contrast (e.g., barium enema) Superficial needle biopsies Clinical laboratory tests requiring arterial puncture Skin biopsies	Over-the-counter drugs Minor surgery with no identified risk factors Physical therapy Occupational therapy IV fluids without additives
Moderate	One or more illnesses with mild exacerbation, progression, or side effects of treatment Two or more stable chronic illnesses Undiagnosed new problem with uncertain prognosis (e.g., lump in breast) Acute illness with systemic symptoms (e.g., pyelonephritis, pneumonitis, colitis) Acute complicated injury (e.g., head injury with brief loss of consciousness)	Physiologic tests under stress (e.g., cardiac stress test, fetal contraction stress test) Diagnostic endoscopies with no identified risk factors Deep needle or incisional biopsy Cardiovascular imaging studies with contrast and no identified risk factors (e.g., arteriogram, cardiac catheterization) Obtain fluid from body cavity (e.g., lumbar puncture, thoracentesis, culdocentesis)	Minor surgery with identified risk factors Elective major surgery (open, percutaneous, or endoscopic) with no identified risk factors Prescription drug management Therapeutic nuclear medicine IV fluids with additives Closed treatment of fracture or dislocation without manipulation
High	One or more chronic illnesses with severe exacerbation, progression, or side effects of treatment Acute or chronic illnesses or injuries that pose a threat to life or bodily function (e.g., multiple trauma, acute MI, pulmonary embolus, severe respiratory distress, progressive severe rheumatoid arthritis, psychiatric illness with potential threat to self or others, peritonitis, acute renal failure) An abrupt change in neurological status (e.g., seizure, TIA, weakness, or sensory loss)	Cardiovascular imaging studies with contrast with identified risk factors Cardiac electrophysiologic tests Diagnostic endoscopies with identified risk factors Discography	Elective major surgery (open, percutaneous, or endoscopic) with identified risk factors Emergency major surgery (open, percutaneous, or endoscopic) Parenteral controlled substances Drug therapy requiring intensive monitoring for toxicity Decision not to resuscitate or to de-escalate care because of poor prognosis

D. Documentation of an Encounter Dominated by Counseling or Coordination of Care

In the case where counseling and/or coordination of care dominates (more than 50%) the physician/patient and/or family encounter (face-to-face time in the office or other outpatient setting, floor/unit time in the hospital or nursing facility), time is considered the key or controlling factor to qualify for a particular level of E/M services.

DG: If the physician elects to report the level of service based on counseling and/or coordination of care, the total length of time of the encounter (face-to-face or floor time, as appropriate) should be documented and the record should describe the counseling and/or activities to coordinate care.

C

Audit Tool

Make multiple copies of the Audit Tool on the next page. Use those copies to help you assign accurate E&M levels to the case studies in Unit 5 and any other time you need to assign an E&M level.

A copy of the Audit Tool and also the E&M Subcategory Questionnaire are available online at http://davisplus.fadavis.com, keyword, Brame.

Professional Charge Audit Worksheet

Patient Name: _____ Provider: _____ DOS: _____

Account Number: _____ Coded: _____ / Audited: _____ Initials: _____

Chief Complaint: _____

HISTORY

History of Present Illness
- ○ Location ○ Quality ○ Timing ○ Modifying factors
- ○ Duration ○ Severity ○ Context ○ Assoc. signs & symptoms

Review of Systems
- ○ Constitut. ○ Cardiovasc. ○ GU ○ Neuro ○ Endocrine
- ○ Eyes ○ Respiratory ○ Musculo ○ Psych ○ Hem/lymph
- ○ ENMT ○ GI ○ Integument (skin, breast) ○ Allerg/imm
- ○ 1 & "All others negative"

Past, Family, Social Histories
- ○ Past (illnesses, operations, allergies, med list)
- ○ Family (family medical history as it pertains to the patient's complaints)
- ○ Social (age-appropriate work, tobacco/alcohol/drugs, school and activities, living situation, etc.)

PHYSICAL EXAM

Organ Systems
- ○ Constitut. ○ Cardiovasc. ○ GU ○ Neuro
- ○ Eyes ○ Respiratory ○ Musculo ○ Psych
- ○ ENMT ○ GI ○ Integument ○ Hem/lymph/imm

Body Areas - *generally use only for major trauma*
- ○ Head ○ Chest ○ Genital/area ○ Left arm ○ Left leg
- ○ Neck ○ Abdomen ○ Back/spine ○ Right arm ○ Right leg
- ○ Unspecified extremity(s)

MEDICAL DECISION MAKING

Diagnosis & Treatment Options (problem is new/est to the provider)

1 Minor problem	X _____	= max 2 _____
1 Established problem, stable or improving	X _____	= _____
2 Established problem, worsening or not improv.	X _____	= _____
3 New problem, no additional work-up planned	X _____	= max 3* _____
4 New problem, additional work-up planned	X _____	= _____

Data to be Reviewed   (listed points, regardless of number of tests)
- 1 Lab order *and/or* review
- 1 Radiology order *and/or* review
- 1 Medicine section of CPT *order and/or* review
- 1 Discuss test results with performing physician
- 1 Decision to obtain old records *and/or* history from someone other than patient
- 2 Review & summary of old records *and/or* obtain hx from non-patient *and/or* discussion of case with another provider
- 2 Personal review of image, tracing, or specimen - not review of report

○ Minimal ○ Low ○ Moderate ○ High
(See Table of Risk)

History Component

HPI	1–3		4+	
ROS	0	1	2–9	10+ or 1+AON
PFSH	0	0	1	2/3*
	PF	EPF	D	C

(Choose marked column farthest to the left)

Exam Component

EXAM	1	2–7L	2–7E	8
	PF	EPF	D	C

Decision Making Component

Diag	1	2	3	4+
Data	0–1	2	3	4+
Risk	Min	Low	Mod	High
	SF	Low	Mod	High

(Choose middle marked column)

OP New/Consults

Hist.	PF	EPF	D	C	C
Exam	PF	EPF	D	C	C
MDM	SF	SF	L	M	H
	1	2	3	4	5

(Choose marked column farthest to the left)

OP Established

Hist.		PF	EPF	D	C
Exam		PF	EPF	D	C
MDM		SF	L	M	H
	1	2	3	4	5

(Choose middle marked column)

Initial Hospital/Obsrv

Hist.	D	C	C
Exam	D	C	C
MDM	L	M	H
	1	2	3

(Choose marked column to the left)

Sub Hospital/Obsrv

Hist.	PF	EPF	D
Exam	PF	EPF	D
MDM	L	M	H
	1	2	3

(Choose middle marked column)

Emergency Department

Hist.	PF	EPF	EPF	D	C
Exam	PF	EPF	EPF	D	C
MDM	SF	L	M	M	H
	1	2	3	4	5

(Choose marked column farthest to the left)

*Complete PFSH: 3 - New OP, Consults, Initial hosp care, hosp observ; 2 - Est OP, Emergency; None - Sub Hosp/Obsrv/NF

Answers to End-of-Chapter Review Questions

■ CHAPTER 1

    1. 4

    2. Annually

    3. 1992

    4. Varies, but should find that the actions are mostly physical.

    5. Varies, but should find that the actions are mostly physical.

    6. Varies, but should find that the actions are mostly mental.

    7. Varies, but should find that the work represented by E&M codes is more concerned with the physician's mental decision making.

    8. Varies

    9. See definitions of *evaluation* and *management*.

  10. Any physician may report any E&M code.

■ CHAPTER 2

    1. One

    2. One

    3. Five

    4. One

    5. Five

    6. The service can be reported.

    7. Not separately reported.

    8. Cannot be determined without knowing the payer—Medicare rules bundle complication care.

    9. The service can be reported.

  10. Cannot be determined without knowing the global period for the procedure.

■ CHAPTER 3

    1. -24

    2. -55

3. -32

4. -25

5. -54, -56

6. -54

7. -56

8. -57

9. -24

10. -32

CHAPTER 4

1. Classification of Evaluation and Management Services, Definitions of Commonly Used Terms, Clinical Examples, and Instructions for Selecting a Level of E&M Service

2. Outpatient

3. Inpatient

4. Patient's relationship to the provider. Patient's medical condition.

5. Type of Service

6. Office or Other Outpatient Services

7. Emergency Department Services

8. Home Services

9. 3

10. Established

CHAPTER 5

1. Outpatient

2. Two of three

3. Many, including physician office, urgent care, hospital-based clinic, hospital outpatient department, emergency department, observation status unit

4. One

5. Inpatient or observation

6. With Same Day Admit Discharge Services

7. Same category as 6

8. C

9. Open 24 hours a day, every day of the year; attached to an acute care facility (hospital)

10. Problem-oriented

CHAPTER 6

1. 30 minutes

2. 99479

3. 29 days to 24 months

4. Critically ill or injured patient and critical care services

5. False

6. 99461

7. 99238

8. 75 minutes

9. 99466

10. The newborn care services codes should not be used for the readmission. The newborn care services describe care provided in the neonate's first admission from delivery to discharge only.

CHAPTER 7

1. Initial Nursing Facility Care

2. Home Services

3. This is not a reported service.

4. Outpatient

5. Nursing facilities are inpatient place of service, and the domiciliary facilities and the patient's home are outpatient places of service.

6. 99315

7. Established to the physician

8. Three questions:

   a. What level of care does the patient receive from the assisted-living community?

   b. If they are in a nursing facility portion of the community, is this an initial or subsequent visit?

   c. If they are in a domiciliary care or private home setting, is the patient new or established to the physician?

9. Consultation

10. Inpatient Consultation

CHAPTER 8

1. Because the time spent in face-to-face prolonged services is always in addition to a base service. Face-to-face prolonged services are never reported on their own.

2. 30 minutes beyond the base code's typical time

3. 90 days

4. 3 INRs

5. 99368

6. 1

7. 99385

8. 99409

9. The next Monday

10. 99455

CHAPTER 9

1. Components

   a. History, examination, medical decision making

   b. Counseling, coordination of care, nature of presenting problem

   c. Time

2. Answers will vary. May not include: Other Emergency Services, Newborn Care, Physician Standby Services, Discharge Services, Telephone Services, Critical Care Services, or Prolonged Physician Direct Services.

3. a. Three of three; b. 99203

4. a. Two of three; b. 99214

5. a. Three of three; b. 99223

6. a. Two of three; b. 99233

7. a. Three of three; b. 99241

8. a. Three of three; b. 99282

9. a. Code specific service; b. 99316

10. a. Code specific service; b. 99377

■ CHAPTER 10

1.

   A. Location

   B. Quality

   C. Severity

   D. Timing

   E. Context

   F. Modifying factors

   G. Associated signs and symptoms

2.

   A. Location

   B. Severity

   C. Context

   D. Quality

   E. Associated signs and symptoms

   F. Modifying factors

   G. Timing

3. Constitutional, Neurological, Musculoskeletal, Cardiovascular, Respiratory, Integumentary, Hematological/lymphatic

4. Constitutional, Eyes, ENMT, Cardiovascular, Respiratory, Integumentary, Neurological, Allergic/Immunological

5.

   A. Past History

   B. ROS

   C. ROS

   D. Past History

   E. Past History

   F. Past History

   G. ROS

   H. ROS

6. Past, Family, and Social History are present.

7. Past and Family History are present.

8. Past History is present. (The fact that the patient has two sisters does not inform the coder about Family or Social History.)

9. Expanded Problem Focused

10. Expanded Problem Focused

▪ CHAPTER 11

 1. Arm (extremity)/Cardiovascular
 2. Abdomen/Gastrointestinal
 3. Abdomen/Immunological
 4. Head/Ears, Nose, Mouth, and Throat
 5. Neck/Ears, Nose, Mouth, and Throat
 6. Chest/Musculoskeletal
 7. Chest/Skin
 8. Genitalia, groin, buttocks/Genitourinary
 9. Back/Musculoskeletal
 10. Leg (extremity)/Musculoskeletal

▪ CHAPTER 12

 1. Moderate Complexity
 2. Low Complexity
 3. High Complexity
 4. Moderate Complexity
 5. Straightforward
 6. Three of three; 99203
 7. Two of three; 99214 (disregard Low Complexity MDM)
 8. Three of three; 99282
 9. Three of three; 99223
 10. Two of three; 99232 (disregard Problem Focused Exam)

▪ CHAPTER 13

 1. 55 minutes (99253)
 2. 25 minutes (99304)
 3. 99202
 4. 99215
 5. 99222
 6. 99231
 7. 99348
 8. Intraservice visit time
 9. Summary of the counseling discussion
 10. That a majority of the visit was spent in counseling and/or coordination of care

▪ CHAPTER 14

 1. History—Comprehensive
 2. History—Detailed
 3. Exam—Comprehensive
 4. Exam—Detailed
 5. MDM—Moderate

6. MDM—Moderate

7.

   a. Office or Other Outpatient

   b. New; affects the level

   c. History—Expanded Problem Focused

      i. Yes

      ii. HPI—Brief

      iii. ROS—Extended

      iv. PFSH—Complete

   d. Exam—Expanded Problem Focused

   e. MDM—Moderate

      i. Number of Diagnoses—3

      ii. Data to Be Reviewed—4

      iii. Risk—Moderate

   f. Three of three

   g. 99202

8.

   a. Initial Hospital Visit

   b. Established; does not apply

   c. History—Comprehensive

      i. Yes

      ii. HPI—Extended

      iii. ROS—Complete

      iv. PFSH—Complete

   d. Exam—Comprehensive

   e. MDM—

      i. Number of Diagnoses: 5 points; 4 for established problem worsening, 1 for established problem stable

      ii. Data to Be Reviewed: 5 points; 1 for Lab, 1 for Radiology, 1 for discussion with performing provider, 2 for discussing the case with another provider

      iii. Risk—Moderate

   f. Three of three

   g. 99222

9.

   a. Office or Other Outpatient

   b. Established; applies

   c. History—Expanded Problem Focused

      i. Yes

      ii. HPI—Brief

      iii. ROS—Problem Pertinent

      iv. PFSH—Pertinent

    d. Exam—Comprehensive

    e. MDM—Moderate

        i. Number of Diagnoses—4

        ii. Data to Be Reviewed—3

        iii. Risk—Moderate

    f. Two of three

    g. 99214

10.

    a. Emergency Department Services

    b. New; does not apply

    c. History—Detailed

        i. Yes

        ii. HPI—Extended

        iii. ROS—Complete

        iv. PFSH—Pertinent

    d. Exam—Detailed

    e. MDM—High

        i. Number of Diagnoses—3

        ii. Data to Be Reviewed—4

        iii. Risk—High

    f. Three of three

    g. 99284

■ CHAPTER 15

1. Detailed

2. Detailed

3. Expanded Problem Focused

4. Seven

5. Four. (There is no Constitutional system element in the Eye Single-System Exam. All other exam notes, regardless of the amount of information provided for each bullet point, count as one bullet point.)

6. Seven

7. Detailed—14 bullet points

8. Eleven

9. Every bullet point in the shaded systems must be listed. At least one bullet point from every unshaded bullet point must be listed. When there is only one bullet point listed, that bullet point must be documented.

10. Every bullet point in the shaded systems must be listed. At least one bullet point from every unshaded bullet point must be listed. When there is only one bullet point listed, that bullet point must be documented.

E

Answers to End-of-Chapter Case Studies

■ CHAPTER 1

1. E&M, Surgery, Radiology, Pathology & Laboratory, Medicine
2. E&M
3. E&M, Surgery
4. Physician's service
5. Not necessarily. The process for selecting professional fee E&M levels and facility E&M levels is very different.

■ CHAPTER 2

1. New patient. Consultations require specific documentation. Any physician can report a consultation, not just specialists.
2. No. Examination headings do not mean anything—only what is documented under them.
3. No. The nephrologist did not make any diagnosis at this visit.
4. No. The nephrologist did not make any diagnosis at this visit. Even though the coder is medically trained, that information cannot be determined for this visit.
5. No. If it was not documented, it was not done.
6. No. Coders do not make medical decisions. If it is documented, it is assumed to be true, accurate, and medically necessary.
7. If the coder has evidence that a service may not have been performed as documented—such as this time discrepancy—the coder should take the information to a supervisor, the office manager, or appropriate compliance professional before determining whether to report the service.

■ CHAPTER 3

1. -25
2. -32
3. -57
4. -54
5. -55
6. -24

CHAPTER 4

1. Dr. Thompson's visit: Place of service, patient status
2. Dr. Singh's category: Type of service
3. Dr. Geld's category: Type of service
4. Dr. Howard's category: Place of service
5. Dr. Thompson's category: Place of service

CHAPTER 5

Internist visit; Office or Other Outpatient Services, Established Patient
Vascular surgeon visit; Consultation Services, Outpatient
Vascular surgeon hospital visit(s); Initial Hospital Services ×1, Subsequent Hospital Services ×3, Inpatient Discharge Day Management ×1
Endocrinologist hospital visit(s); Consultation Services, Inpatient ×1, Subsequent Hospital Services ×3
Vascular surgeon follow-up visit; Office or Other Outpatient Services, Established Patient
Internist follow-up visit; Office or Other Outpatient Services, Established Patient

CHAPTER 6

Neonatologist code(s), if applicable:
Day 1: 99468, 99464, 31500
Day 2: 99469
Day 3: 99469
Day 4: 99469
Day 5: 99469
Day 6: 99469
Day 7: 99469
Neonatologist code(s) at Grace Hospital, if applicable: None
Neonatologist code(s) in transport, if applicable: 99466, 99467
Neonatal pulmonologist code(s), if applicable: 99468
Neonatal pulmonologist code(s), if applicable:
Day 9: 99469
Day 10: 99469
Day 11: 99469
Day 12: 99469
Day 13: 99469
Day 14: 99469
Day 15: 99469
Day 16: 99478
Day 17: 99478
Day 18: 99479
Day 19: 99479
Day 20: 99479
Day 21: 99479
Day 22: 99479
Day 23: 99479
Day 24: 99479
Day 25: 99479
Neonatal pulmonologist code(s), if applicable:
Day 45: Subsequent hospital care codes 99231–99233
Day 53: 99238

CHAPTER 7

1. Hospital Discharge Services
2. Initial Nursing Facility Care
3. Subsequent Nursing Facility Care
4. Subsequent Nursing Facility Care
5. Inpatient Consultation
6. No reportable services. The patient was not admitted or discharged.
7. Not a separately reported service. The patient was not admitted or discharged.
8. Part of the global surgical package.
9. Other Nursing Facility Services
10. Inpatient Consultation—A physician may report a consultation every time an opinion is requested, even if the patient is established to the practice.
11. Nursing Facility Discharge Services
12. No reported service
13. Domiciliary, Rest Home (e.g., Boarding Home), or Custodial Care Services, Established Patient
14. Domiciliary, Rest Home (e.g., Assisted Living Facility), or Home Care Plan Oversight Services

CHAPTER 8

1. Preventive Medicine Services, New Patient
2. Telephone Services
3. No reportable service because the patient did not initiate the service, and it was within 7 days of another call
4. Face-to-face prolonged services
5. Non–face-to-face prolonged services
6. Medical team conference
7. Care Plan Oversight Services, Home Health
8. Work Related or Medical Disability Evaluation Services

CHAPTER 9

1. 99284
2. 99202
3. 99202
4. 99254
5. 99203
6. 99214
7. 99385

CHAPTER 10

1. Foreign object in eye
2. Location (eye); Context (while at work welding); Associated signs and symptoms (pain, light-headedness, shortness of breath); Severity (pain is 8 on a 10-point scale)
3. Extended (4 elements)

4. Constitutional; Eye (vision is blurred); ENMT (mouth feels dry); Cardiovascular (heart is racing); Respiratory (shortness of breath); Gastrointestinal (not nauseated); Musculoskeletal (no pain in head or neck); Integumentary (no debris in face or arms); Neurological (no headache)

5. Eye

6. Problem-pertinent and limited additional systems (9 systems, Eye + 8 additional systems)

7. Past (No surgical history; Previous history of splinter in eye; NKDA; No daily medications); Social (Patient lives alone)

8. Pertinent (Complete requires all three history types)

9. Detailed (Chief Complaint, Extended HPI, Problem-pertinent and limited additional systems ROS, Pertinent PFSH)

■ CHAPTER 11

1. Body areas
   a. Head (eyes, eyelids, nares, face)
   b. Neck (no foreign bodies)
   c. Chest (respirations, heart rate)
   d. Extremities × 2 (no foreign bodies in hands)

2. Organ system
   a. Eye
   b. Ears, Nose, Mouth, Throat
   c. Skin (no foreign bodies, not diaphoretic)
   d. Cardiovascular
   e. Respiratory

3. Either body areas or organ systems is acceptable, as long as the student has sound reasoning for the answer. Body area could be more appropriate because the patient presents with trauma, and care is focused on the head as a body area. Organ systems may be more appropriate because care is focused on the eye.

4. Detailed. Multiple eye structures and additional organ systems are examined. This could also be determined by ruling out other levels. The eye exam is not limited, so the lower levels do not apply. A general multisystem exam was not performed (assuming this means all systems are examined), and a complete single system exam was not performed (all major eye structures are not noted), so a comprehensive exam does not apply.

■ CHAPTER 12

Case Study 1
1. Multiple
2. Minimal or None
3. Moderate
4. Amount and/or Complexity of Data to Be Reviewed
5. Moderate Complexity

Case Study 2
1. Emergency Department Services
2. N/A
3. Three of three
4. 99284

Case Study 3

1. Office or Other Outpatient Services

2. New

3. Borderline glucose levels

4. Timing (1 month ago), Context (found as a result of the hospital stay, increases after eating), Severity (never exceeded 200 mg/dl), Associated Signs and Symptoms (frequent urination), Modifying factors (diet and exercise)

5. Extended (five elements of HPI)

6. Constitutional, Eye, Hematological, Neurological, ENMT, Integumentary, GU, GI, Cardiovascular, Respiratory, Musculoskeletal, Psychiatric, Endocrine, Allergic/Immunological

7. Endocrine

8. All systems reviewed

9. Past, Family, and Social Histories

10. Complete

11. Comprehensive

12. Head, Neck, Chest, Abdomen, Genitalia, Extremities ×4

13. Eyes, ENMT, Cardiovascular, Respiratory, Gastrointestinal, Genitourinary, Musculoskeletal, Skin, Neurological, Psychiatric, Hematological/lymphatic/immunological

14. This is not a trauma, so organ systems would probably be more appropriate.

15. Because the physician examined all organ systems recognized by CPT, the exam is comprehensive.

16. Multiple

17. Moderate

18. Moderate

19. All three are the same level; any could be chosen as "lowest"

20. Moderate complexity

21. Three of three

22. Comprehensive, Comprehensive, Moderate

23. 99204

■ CHAPTER 13

1. 99202
2. 99203
3. 99251
4. 99204 (Do not include non–face-to-face time in the office.)

■ CHAPTER 14

1. Office or Other Outpatient
2. New; applies
3. History—Comprehensive
   a. Borderline glucose levels
   b. HPI—Extended
   c. ROS—Complete
   d. PFSH—Complete
4. Exam—Comprehensive

5. MDM—Low

   a. Number of Diagnoses—3

   b. Data to Be Reviewed—1

   c. Risk—Low

6. Three of three

7. 99203

■ CHAPTER 15

1. General Multi-System Exam is best.

2. Total bullet points—21

3. Total systems with at least one bullet point—11

4. Total systems with at least two bullet points—3

5. Detailed Exam type—12 elements from at least two systems. A Comprehensive Exam type is not met because while there are nine systems noted, there are not at least two bullet points noted in each.

6. The 1995 Guidelines. The 1995 Exam was Comprehensive, which is higher than the 1997 Guidelines Detailed Exam.

   a. Head: normocephalic, atraumatic

      i. 1 bullet point, **musculoskeletal** inspection of the head

   b. Neck: supple, trachea midline, no lymphadenopathy

      i. 1 bullet point, **neck** examination of the neck

      ii. 1 bullet point, **lymph** palpation of neck

   c. Eyes: grossly normal

      i. No bullet point, not specific enough

   d. ENMT: mucous membranes pink

      i. 1 bullet point, **ENMT** inspection of nasal mucosa

      ii. 1 bullet point, **ENMT** inspection of oral mucosa

   e. Cardiovascular: RRR

      i. 1 bullet point, **cardiovascular** auscultation of heart

   f. Respiratory: clear breath sounds bilateral

      i. 1 bullet point, **respiratory** auscultation of lungs

   g. GI: Positive bowel sounds, no organomegaly

      i. No bullet point, not specific enough

   h. GU: external genitalia normal, no hernias palpated

      i. 1 bullet point, **GU male** examination of the penis

      ii. 1 bullet point, **gastrointestinal** examination for hernia

   i. Extremities: full ROM in all four extremities; positive reflexes and strength × 4; no skin changes noted

      i. 4 bullet points, **musculoskeletal** assessment of range of motion, all four extremities

      ii. 4 bullet points, **musculoskeletal** assessment of muscle strength, all four extremities

      iii. 1 bullet point, **neurological** examination of deep tendon reflexes

      iv. 1 bullet point, **skin** inspection of skin

   j. Neuro: cranial nerves II–XII normal; patient is oriented × 3

      i. 1 bullet point, **neurological** test cranial nerves

      ii. 1 bullet point, **psychiatric** brief assessment of mental status, including orientation

Glossary

Add-on code: CPT codes that are only reported in addition to another CPT code.

All others negative (AON): An abbreviation when all systems are reviewed and the non–problem pertinent systems are negative.

AMA: American Medical Association—The AMA publishes the Current Procedural Terminology annually, which includes the codes reported for Evaluation and Management services.

Ambulatory care: Patient receiving services but not confined to the hospital.

ARNP: Advanced Registered Nurse Practitioner—An ARNP is a Registered Nurse (RN) with advanced training who may see patients independently from a physician.

Assessment: Consists of the process used in order to arrive at a diagnosis.

Assisted living facilities: Similar to nursing facilities in that they provide room and board and personal assistance services, but they do not include a nursing service component.

Auscultation: The act of listening to a part of the body.

Care plan oversight: Management of all patient services without face-to-face services. May include a variety of services including time spent reviewing patient status reports, laboratory and other diagnostic study results, adjusting medical therapy, and communication with other health care professionals, family members, surrogate decision makers, and caregivers regarding assessment of the patient and decisions regarding care.

Chief complaint: Patient's presenting problem, the foundation of every E&M note.

CNM: Certified Nurse Midwife—A CNM is a nurse with advanced training in midwifery, including pre-natal care, delivery, and post-natal care of both mother and baby.

Consult 3 Rs: Request, Render, Report.

Contributing components: CPT defined components that often exist but are not necessary to a note—Counseling, Coordination of Care, Nature of Presenting Problem.

Coordination of care: Contributing component that includes ordering diagnostic studies, planning return visits, asking a nurse to complete incidental care, and other associated services.

Counseling: Contributing component that describes the physician discussing with the patient diagnosis and treatment options.

Critical care services: A physician's constant attention to one patient with a high level of effort to diagnose and treat the patient.

Critically ill or injured patient: Patient that has suffered significant impairment to at least one vital organ system or is at imminent risk of such impairment.

Consultation: A medical professional is asked for an opinion regarding a patient's diagnosis or how best to treat a patient's condition.

CPT: Current Procedural Terminology—CPT is published annually by the American Medical Association, including the codes for reporting Evaluation & Management services.

Diagnosis: The underlying cause of symptoms, the nature of an illness.

Duration: How long the patient has had the chief complaint.

Elements: Building blocks of a Key Component.

Emergency Department: An Emergency Department is accessible 24 hours a day, every day of the year, and is physically attached to an acute care facility, in the event a patient needs a higher level of care.

Established patient: A patient who has received services from the physician within the past 3 years.

Evaluation: The physician effort of forming an opinion about the patient's condition. Determining something systematically.

Evaluation and Management: The act of diagnosing and treating an illness or injury, not including performing procedures or testing that can be reported with a CPT code from another chapter.

Exam: Key component that describes the objective portion of the visit.

Face-to-face: Working in the physical presence of the patient. For hospital visits, also time spent on the unit/floor dedicated to the patient.

Freestanding: Not attached to a hospital facility.

Global surgical package: When a surgery or other major procedure is performed, the CPT code reported for the surgery refers to more than the surgery alone. The surgical CPT code represents an inclusive package of services covering all the relevant elements of the surgery, such as local anesthesia and immediate post-operative care.

History: Key component that describes the subjective portion of the visit.

History of present illness (HPI): The story of the patient's chief complaint from the first signs of the condition to the current visit or from the last time the patient saw the physician for the condition to the current visit.

Home: A private residence with no coordinated care services.

Hospital inpatient facilities: Facilities that provide nursing care for patients with acute illness or injury.

HPI—Brief: 1-3 elements of HPI.

HPI—Extended: 4 or more elements of HPI.

Inpatient: Specific admit status to a hospital or nursing facility.

Inspection: A variety of ways in which the physician visualizes or observes the patient's anatomy and body habitus.

Intraservice time: Time spent face-to-face with the patient.

Key components: CPT defined note components that are the basic building blocks of a note—History, Exam, and Medical Decision Making.

Legible: As least one of three reviewers must be able to read the note.

Management: The physician effort of determining an appropriate treatment course for the patient's condition. The treatment of disease or injury.

Management options: Documentation of the plan portion of the visit.

Medical decision making (MDM): Key component that describes the assessment and plan portions of the visit.

Medical necessity: Concept closely related to Nature of Presenting Problem, relating to whether the services rendered were necessary to treat the patient's condition effectively.

Medicare Physician Fee Schedule Database: MPFSDB provides the information used by Medicare as a basis to determine payment. The file contains the associated relative value units, a fee schedule status indicator, and modifiers.

Modifiers: Modifiers further describe an E/M service that has been altered due to the situation in which the services were provided, but modifiers do not change the definition of the underlying CPT code.

Nature of presenting problem: Contributing component that is much more of a conceptual component, describing how many differential diagnoses a presenting problem creates, or the typical outcome for a presenting problem.

Neonatologist: Physician specializing in newborn care and related diseases.

New patient: A patient who has not received services from the provider of the current service within the last 3 years.

Newborn: Patient aged 0–28 days.

Non–face-to-face: Work that is not in the physical presence of the patient.

Nurse visit: Visit in which the patient sees a nurse only, without seeing a physician.

Nursing facilities: Facilities that provide care for patients still in need of monitored nursing care, but who no longer require care for acute illness or injury.

Objective: Observing the patient through examination.

Obstetrician: Physician specializing in pregnancy, birth, and maternal care.

One rule: The premise that a physician may report one E&M code per day for each patient seen. One Physician, One code, One day.

OPPS: Medicare reimburses hospital facilities for outpatient services based on the Outpatient Prospective Payment System.

Outpatient: A patient who is specifically not an inpatient in a hospital or nursing facility.

Oversight services: One or more providers involved in the patient's care reviewing data, communicating regarding the patient's condition or care, and making further care decisions.

PA: Physician Assistants practice medicine under the supervision of a physician.

Palpation: Touching the body.

Past, family, social history (PFSH):   Describes the patient's history and environmental factors that might cause or affect the chief complaint or influence the patient's recovery.

Patient status: The patient's physical condition or the patient's relationship to the provider.

Percussion: Tapping a body part and listening to the result.

PFSH—Complete: 2 or 3 history types, depending on E&M category.

PFSH—Pertinent: 1 history type, past, family or social.

Place of service: Physical location requirement for the services rendered.

Plan: Determining how to manage the diagnosis or a plan for further testing to determine a diagnosis.

Postpartum: Immediately following delivery.

Practice group: Payers consider all providers in the same specialty practice group to be one entity when it comes to payment.

Pre-existing condition: Condition that was present prior to the current treatment.

Presenting problem: The reason for the visit.

Preventive medicine services: Physician service to prevent disease. Patient presents without specific complaint.

Principal component: Time becomes the overwhelming factor for the visit when counseling and coordination of care are the majority of the visit.

Problem-oriented: Visit to treat a patient with a presenting problem, as opposed to preventive care.

Procedures: Physician services are generally divided into procedures and visits. Procedures are therapeutic or diagnostic actions performed on the patient.

Professional coding: Professional coding is the practice of determining the appropriate codes to report for services rendered by healthcare professionals, rather than facility coding.

Qualified Health Professional: As defined in the CPT introduction, "An individual who is qualified by education, training, licensure/regulation (when applicable), and facility privileging (when applicable) who performs a professional service within his/her scope of practice and independently reports that professional service."

Qualitative: Measured by descriptive terms.

Quantitative: Measured by the amount of information documented.

Referral: Recommendation to another medical provider without necessarily receiving any information in return.

Render: Documentation of a consultation visit.

Report: Evidence the consulting physician sent a written report to the requesting physician.

Request: Notation that a requestor has asked the consulting physician some question about a patient's condition and/or treatment options.

Review of systems (ROS):   The physician asks questions to determine whether the patient has any other issues that might affect the chief complaint. Recorded by organ system.

ROS—Complete: 10-14 systems reviewed.

ROS—Extended: 2-9 systems reviewed.

ROS—Problem pertinent: 1 system reviewed.

SOAP note: Documentation format taught in medical school.

Structured screening: A pre-conceived screening method to assess a patient condition.

Subcategories: Divisions of an E&M section.

Subjective: Consists of asking the patient questions.

Surgical package: When a surgery or other major procedure is performed, the CPT code reported for the surgery refers to more than the surgery alone. The surgical CPT code represents an inclusive package of services covering all the relevant elements of the surgery, such as anesthesia and immediate post-operative care. Also known as global surgical package.

Time: Seventh component; the length of the E&M service.

Transfer of care: The requesting physician sends the patient for a specific treatment or has determined a diagnosis and refers the patient for whatever treatment the specialist concludes is needed, but does not ask a question of the specialist.

Type of service: A particular service being provided, such as Consultations.

Underlying condition: Condition which caused need for the treatment, but which is not resolved by the treatment.

Visit: Physician services are generally divided into procedures and visits. Visits comprise physician mental effort to evaluate and manage the patient's condition.

INDEX

Page numbers followed by b indicate box
Page numbers followed by f indicate figure
Page numbers followed by t indicate table